ROSE FLOWER ESSENCES

A New Guide to Natural Healing
With 65 Remedies
Made From
The World's Most Beloved Flower

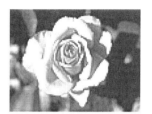

ROSE FLOWER ESSENCES

A New Guide to Natural Healing
With 65 Remedies
Made From
The World's Most Beloved Flower

BY
Tenanche Rose Golden, M.A., R.M.T.
Rosaflora Flower Essences

Cover Design: Angi Shearstone
www.angishearstone.com
Interior Layout: integrative ink
www.integrativeink.com
Editor: Judith Burnett Schneider
www.fatplum.com
Front Cover Photo: © Eric M. Renard
www.renardadv.com
Back Cover and Interior Photos: © Collette Morton
www.tucsonrose.org

Includes bibliographic references and index.
ISBN 1-4116-6056-0
LCCN 2005939083

Printed in the United States of America

Published by
Healing Rose Press
P.O. Box 91104
Pittsburgh, PA 15221

DEDICATION

This book is lovingly dedicated to my parents,

Dr. Marion L. Poole
(1921-2000)
and
Dr. Rachel J. Poole

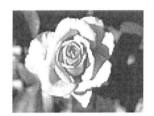

A Special Thank You To:

God - Father, Son, and Holy Spirit
Loving Creator of the magnificent plant kingdom and the healing
signature of the rose.
Thank you for loving me and for placing a deep love of roses into
my heart.

Cinde Sevey
For allowing me to prepare my first flower essence in your desert
herb garden many years ago.

Sandy Miller and Melva Wheeler
For your expertise and guidance in organic rose gardening and
nearly endless supply of roses for research.

Collette Morton
For spending time in the rose garden with me to take your
beautiful photos of the roses.

Ørjan Repaal
For contributing your valuable clinical observations of the rose
flower essences to this research.

All of you who have participated in the Rose Essence Research
Program and the Biofeedback Imaging Sessions:
You have provided valuable information that contributes to the
field of flower essence therapy.

Donna Crystal
Biofeedback imaging technician extraordinaire.

Judith Burnett Schneider
For your expert critique and enthusiastic suggestions during the
final manuscript edit.

Stephanee Killen and her staff at *integrative ink*
For your patience and professionalism
during the interior formatting.

Angi Shearstone
For the beautiful cover layout and design.

Eric Renard
For the exquisite cover photo.

Jeannine Lanigan, Stephanie Simmons, and Ziporah Hildebrandt
For slogging through the first versions of the manuscript
seemingly eons ago.
Thanks for your input.

Matomah Alesha of Matam Press and Sandra Gould Ford of
Radiant Tree
For all of your publishing advice and support.

Adriene and M
For your loving encouragement and for being the best sisters in
the world.

Richard Johnson
For believing in me and in this project and
for your financial support.

Aunt Bernice, my nieces Aisha and Jonolyn and my nephew E.J.
and brother-in-law Tim
You have been an inspiration and a blessing to me.

Joy Goodheart, Estela Parke, Elaine Robinson, A.L.

For hanging in with me through the ups and downs of life and in writing this book.

Mom and Dad
Your guidance and support have positively impacted my life. Because of your love, sacrifice and commitment to excellence, this book has become a reality.

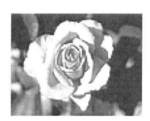

CONTENTS

INTRODUCTION

How beautiful you are, fragrant rose!
Oh, how your dew heals my heart!

$\mathcal{R}$ ose flower essences are natural heart-healing remedies. They are truly gifts from God!

This book focuses on the distinct possibilities of healing the heart and soul when one uses the essences of the Rose, the Universal Flower of Love. Rose flower essences can help to balance us emotionally and spiritually, stabilize our nervous system and support our immune system. The essences of this beloved flower can inspire us to appreciate the profound and magnificent beauty of God's creation, to move into states of love, joy, devotion and celebration.

As I have been writing this book, I have wondered how it would be different from the many other books on flower essences out there today. I am pleased to say that there are a few similarities as well as some major differences.

You'll find that this is the first book that focuses exclusively on rose flower essences. Other books on flower essences include only a limited number of roses among many other flowers. Through my research I have found that rose flower essences offer a unique healing system. This system is a branching of the healing quality of the *Wild Rose* flower essence discovered by British physician, Dr. Edward Bach, creator of the Bach Flower Remedies during the 1930s. This healing system helps to address the stress, emotional and spiritual issues we face in the 21st century.

Secondly, you'll find that there is a "poetry of healing" offered by these wonderful remedies that comes through in their healing descriptions. As I've meditated and contemplated while taking essences and spending time with and observing the roses in the organic garden over many weeks, months and now years, many healing words have come to inspire and nurture me during the process. These poetic messages have supported me through many personal challenges: separation, divorce, job-related stress, change of jobs, the passing of my father, and relocation from the beautiful Arizona desert to the rolling hills of Pennsylvania. By helping me to deepen my self-awareness and nurture my heart, these inspiring words and healing essences have been uplifting to my spirit and soothing to my soul.

The messages take form in the beautiful quotes that precede the descriptions of the rose flower essence formulas, which combine the healing energies of roses and other flowers. As you use the essences daily, these healing words offer comfort, encouragement and support. You may be awed and amazed at the spiritual inspirations that you will experience while using rose flower essences: subtle, yet powerful emissaries of healing and love in liquid form.

In this book, there are anecdotal case stories and testimonials from those who have used the essences, including clinical case examples offered by homeopath-homotoxicologist, Ørjan Repaal of the ABC klinikken in Oslo, Norway as well as excerpts from a 7-week journal by a LaStone Therapy™ massage therapist who shares her experiences. These observations of the benefits experienced by many users of the rose flower essences provide testimony of the gentle healing support that these remedies offer.

Books on flower essences have traditionally offered repertories full of single flower essence profiles, their benefits and the personality imbalances they affect. You will find that here also, as there are descriptions of 52 individual rose flower essences and

13 combination formulas, their healing potentials, the imbalances they address and applications for them.

In Chapter Nine, you are encouraged to make your own essences by acquiring the roses and flowers in the wild or from your own organic garden. Along with the practical application of the rose essences, the organic rose garden and the outdoors play a major role in the healing process. You will be able to integrate your own organic garden or natural surroundings as venues for creative, growth-inspiring activities in conjunction with using the essences to further facilitate natural healing on a deep level. Chapter Four details current research that provides evidence that viewing and spending time in a natural garden can accelerate healing.

This book suggests ways to use the rose flower essences other than by taking them by mouth. A chapter on using the essences in bath therapy lists essences for aroma-massage (aromatherapy combined with massage therapy) and a chart of body energy centers suggests areas for topical healing applications.

There are several natural healing modalities that will support your healing work with the essences. Massage, Rolfing, somatic therapies, breath therapies, meditation, contemplation, prayer, journaling, dance, movement and play are among them. You'll find a list of contact information to locate qualified practitioners and teachers of these modalities included at the end of the book.

Appendix B includes a chart that correlates 16 roses with their corresponding combination formulas to help you find the rose flower essence you seek. There are also charts that describe the original fragrance of each rose blossom (there is no fragrance present in the rose flower essence itself) and its corresponding body application points to help you in the selection process.

For those with more scientific leanings, this book discusses research on Vitamin C, a nutrient in rose hips, and its compelling connections to healing with rose flower essences. The chapter on biofeedback imaging photography sessions that confirm changes in the human bio-energy field and energy centers in conjunction with taking the rose flower essences offers compelling evidence for their healing and balancing properties. Crystallography, and the phenomenon called "the memory of water" are also discussed to further ground the information about flower essence therapy into the realm of sub-molecular science.

I hope that, as you explore this book, you will gain more understanding and experience in this exciting and fascinating field of natural healing. I sincerely hope that you find this book informative, supportive, and uplifting as well as a helpful companion for you on your natural healing journey with rose flower essences.

Tenanche Rose Golden, M.A., R.M.T.
March, 2005

CHAPTER 1
FLOWER ESSENCES:
TOOLS FOR HEALING

What are flower essences?
How do they work?
How are they made?
Will they work for me?

*F*lower essences are all-natural remedies made from the flower's blossom rather than from its leaves or roots, as herbal extracts are made. While taking herbal remedies can affect us physically, using flower essences can help us to manage the emotional and psychological stresses that we face in life. They can also help us to overcome emotional and mental limitations, increase wellbeing and inspire us to reach our God-given potential.

Flower essences are natural healing agents. A flower essence is a potent liquid infusion that holds the energy imprint or *signature* of a flower blossom within the molecular structure of water. The infusion has no fragrance as does an essential oil. When taken by mouth or applied to points on the body, this infusion carries the plant's unique healing qualities to the user without any physical evidence of the flower being present within it.

Flower essences are not drugs. They do not work in the same way as anti-depressants or tranquilizers or even aspirin from your local pharmacy. They are safe to use because they are non-toxic and do not react chemically within the body, as do prescription drugs. Their effect is, instead, bio-energetic. They work on the physical-mental-emotional body by helping to balance subtle energy systems rather than by suppressing symptoms and driving them deeper into the body.

Much like homeopathic remedies, flower essences can catalyze a noticeable physical, mental or emotional healing effect immediately or over time. The healing effect is more likely to be sustained with no side effects because it is caused by the body's own natural healing response.

Historical Uses of Flower Essences

Though considered a "new" science, the therapeutic use of flower essences dates back some ten thousand years. The earliest known tradition was among the aboriginal people of Australia. Research has validated the use of flower remedies in their ceremonial practices and flower saunas which are still practiced today.[1] A tradition of flower essence therapy in Malaysia and Thailand, where temples specialize in flower essence healing, is also still in practice.[2] In Native American, African, Polynesian cultures and virtually every indigenous culture in the world, the life-force of a plant is believed to be the most concentrated in its flowers. The flower blossom is considered to be a powerful healing agent.[3]

Flower Essence Therapy in the West

Dr. Edward Bach, a British bacteriologist and homeopath, was one of the first modern pioneers of healing with flower essences. He is credited with introducing the therapy to western medicine during the first half of the 20th century. Through his meticulous research between the years 1930 and 1936, Dr. Bach introduced 38 basic flower remedies to the western world. He discovered that flower essences helped the body to heal itself by working with its vital essence or *life-force* energy. He also found that these remedies worked by balancing the emotions and mental attitudes that were the underlying causes of physical diseases. Through thousands of case studies gathered over the years, these remedies have proven to be so effective that the U.S. Food and Drug Administration approves them.

The Bach Flower Remedies, and especially, the Rescue Remedy™, can be found in virtually every health-food store in the world. Because of their supportive role in healing, thousands of registered Bach practitioners and holistic health professionals incorporate these and other flower essences into their practices.

Why Use Rose Flower Essences?

The healing energies in rose flower essences uniquely influence the body's subtle energy systems. Rose flower essences can help us to balance and harmonize our emotions, where negative emotional and mental attitudes have contributed to illness. In a non-invasive way, they can also help to clear away the limiting emotional and mental patterns that keep us from being and living to our full potential. They are a great complementary therapy to any holistic health enhancement program that may include daily exercise, balanced diet, stress reduction, personal and spiritual development, and holistic health care.

Should I Take Rose Flower Essences?

Hmm, sounds good, you say. *Maybe I'll run out and buy a rose flower essence, slip a few drops into hubby's morning brew and put a check on his annoying habits.*

That may seem like a good idea, but flower essences tend to work best when we willingly choose and responsibly work with them ourselves. They can gently bring to our conscious awareness the fragmented and broken areas within us that need nurturing and support, and help us to move toward emotional and mental harmony.

Rose flower essences aren't for everybody. People with severe mental and emotional imbalances shouldn't take flower essences unless under the strict supervision of a qualified professional experienced in using flower essences with other forms of therapy. Anyone who is committed to working on personal and spiritual growth would benefit by using rose flower essences. Children and animals and even plants are far more open to natural healing than adults and they usually respond to them very well.

How Do I Choose and Take a Rose Flower Essence?

If you feel that you might benefit from rose flower essences, you can easily make your own. Directions for making them can be found in Chapter Nine. You can also obtain ready-to-use flower essences from many companies and retail outlets, at local health-food stores or on the Internet and add them to your own personal healing program.

If you're curious about which of the essences in this book might benefit you, there are various testing and diagnostic tools, such as kinesiology (muscle checking—a type of body biofeedback) and self and practitioner assessment.

Chapter Seven offers basic instructions on using kinesiology for choosing flower essences to support your healing. You can also use keywords, such as *self-serving* or *compassionate,* that suggest imbalances addressed by, or the healing potential of each essence or formula. These are included in the descriptions of the combination formulas and in the Rose Flower Essence Repertory and in lists at the back of the book.

When taking your flower essence, take 1–2 drops of a stock essence, which is a more concentrated version, under the tongue or sip in pure water or juice. In the case of a dosage essence, which is a dilution of the stock essence, take about 4 drops to a full dropper under your tongue. While taking essences, refrain from using caffeine, tobacco, alcohol, illegal drugs and other toxic substances (such as overly-processed or preserved foods) that interfere or suppress the body's own innate healing processes. Flower essences can be applied externally to pulse points and energy centers on the body. They can be used in bath therapy and can be mist sprayed around your body and in your environment.

CHAPTER 2
ROSE PARADIGMS:
HEALING WITH ROSE FLOWER ESSENCES

*H*ow many times have you felt that you might become "unglued" in the face of sudden change, trauma, a personal loss or even an overwhelming event? As you will see, rose flower essences can help you to stay centered, endure and nurture yourself when you most need it. They can help to lend courage and perseverance and provide the resilience you need to carry on.

A Brief History of the Rose

The rose has a popular legacy crossing many world cultures. For thousands of years, the beauty and fragrance of the rose has been treasured the world over. Among many cultures rich mythologies and symbolisms are associated with the rose, a testament to this flower's universal appeal.

The rose is a universal symbol of the qualities of love, divine beauty and grace. It can also represent deep passion and desire. With these spiritual and nurturing qualities, it is no wonder we love to connect with one another by exchanging roses!

The Persians are credited for cultivating the first garden rose. Roses, of course, had been growing in the wild long before in the Orient. The western world is probably indebted to the Chinese for introducing the original wild roses. These wild, or "species" roses were the distant ancestors of the modern long-stemmed, hybrid tea roses so familiar to us today.

There are so many more rose types or varieties. Among them are the damasks and gallicas—the "old garden" roses that pre-date the first hybrid tea roses (bred in 1867) and date back to ancient Roman and Persian gardens. Chinese gardens were adorned with small, tender repeat-blooming roses before 300 B.C! [1]

Presently, there are well over 5,000 varieties of hybridized roses (also known as cultivars) and more are being introduced to commerce everyday. All are descendents of the original wild, species roses and display a wide range of colors, sizes, number of petals and variety of fragrances that range from sweet to apple, musk, pepper and even tea.

Why the Rose?

The rose is the most universally recognized and beloved flower in the world. Various interpretations and symbolisms connected with roses depend on the color and fragrance of each individual rose. (See Appendix A)

Roses are no strangers to the art of healing. They've been used for centuries all over the world as medicinal tonics to help cure ailments, as mood enhancers, in cosmetics, perfumes, as aphrodisiacs, and even as culinary additives. Of course, they also add beauty and grace to gardens, homes and workspaces.

In many parts of the world it's customary to give roses as a token of one's love, affection and devotion. When a person is ill, roses are brought to them to uplift and comfort them with their beautiful colors, exquisite fragrances and healing vibrations.

We often exchange roses at transitional life-events such as birth, congratulatory moments, romance, marriage and anniversaries, and even in illness and death. We humans intuitively know that this is one of the rose's healing signatures: to support us through many transitions and evolutionary processes in life. [2]

6

Roses and Their Essences as Therapeutic Aids

The ingestion of roses for therapeutic purposes has been documented in many cultures throughout history.

In Ayurvedic medical practices in India, the tea of *Rosa damascena* has been used as a laxative, blood purifier and tonic to the digestive and reproductive organs.[3]

Among the Romans there was a tradition of using *Rosa gallica* to treat 32 conditions, ranging from stomach ache and insomnia to purification of the mind and strengthening the heart.[4]

Rose hips, high in Vitamin C, have been used in folk remedies and teas for conditions such as constipation, kidney and bladder problems, and exhaustion. The hip is the bright red ovary or seed-filled "fruit" of the rose, about the size of a cherry, which remains after the rose petals have fallen off. It contains flavenoids, which increase the body's use of the Vitamin C contained in the hip, itself. Rose hips are considered to be the most potent natural source of Vitamin C known today.[5]

Vitamin C and Lycopene, a carotene also found in roses, are both antioxidants which are known to combat stress, nervousness, heart disease, cancer and help to maintain a healthy immune system.[6] These nutrients are supportive to the immune system, which protects the body from invasion by unhealthy organisms.

The rose has been used traditionally as a medicinal agent in the form of rosewater (an excellent healing tonic for skin cells), rose essential oil, ointments, salves, teas, perfumes and fragrances the world over.

Rose Flower Essences as a Branched Healing System

The blossom of a rose makes a very effective flower essence. According the Dr. Edward Bach, founder of the Bach Flower Remedies in the 1930s, the flower essence of *Wild Rose* is a remedy for healing the personality imbalance of apathy or resignation to one's circumstances. In this case scenario, the person just gives up on finding any joy or purpose in life, resigning himself to life's struggles. *Wild Rose* essence helps to bring a person back to living a life of enthusiasm, pleasure and joy.[7] Since Dr. Bach's discovery thousands of practitioners and self-care users have confirmed this healing quality of *Wild Rose* flower essence.

The wild rose is also known as a *species rose*. This rose has not been crossbred with another rose. Dr. Bach used the species *Rosa canina* to make his remedy and discovered its healing benefits. During several years of research with essences made from cultivated roses, I have found that flower essences made from cross-bred (hybridized) roses also offer healing benefits. This demonstrates a branching of the rose's healing qualities among hybridized garden-grown roses.

For example, while the *Wild Rose* flower essence specifically addresses resignation in the personality and cultivates pleasure and joy, as outlined by Dr. Bach, certain cultivated or garden-grown roses address the imbalance by supporting a broader range of positive soul qualities. A specific rose or group of roses can support the opening and healing of the heart, bringing forth positive soul qualities such as self-acceptance, compassion, and self-nurture. The personality may then begin to become aware of spiritual aspirations, such as gratitude, compassion and forgiveness, among many others. I have experienced this process myself, as have many clients who have used the rose flower essences.

Thus, with the hybridization of roses, I believe that the healing potential of the rose has expanded since Dr. Bach's time. Rose flower essences present a healing system that can help us to address the emotional needs and spiritual challenges of our times.

The Healing Signature of the Rose

The healing signature, or blueprint of each rose cultivar can be found within the characteristics of each rose variety: its thorns,

8

the bloom (petals and color and fragrance), the hips and in the plant's hardiness. We can see parallels between the physical qualities and nutrients in the plant and the emotional qualities it helps to balance.

For instance, the many thorns on the rose stem symbolize repeated painful life experiences. In humans, at the emotional level, pain is experienced in one's heart center, which is located next to the thymus gland – a chief agent of the immune system.

The hips of the rose contain nutrients, like Vitamin C and Lycopene, that support the heart and the immune system, which protects the body from invasion by unhealthy organisms.

The rose flower essence, with a healing signature connected with these nutrients, affects one at the emotional level. It soothes and balances the nervous system and supports and protects the heart from emotional pain and trauma.[8] This flower essence also fosters hardiness, resilience and endurance in the face of sudden changes, characteristics that all repeat-blooming rose cultivars tend to display after being pruned.

By taking a rose flower essence, one who has experienced hurt and trauma may find comfort, be sustained and fortified. More able to emotionally bounce back after being cut down, they may find it easier to deal with the unexpected challenges of life.

The Positive Soul Qualities Supported
By Rose Flower Essences

A rose flower essence, then, helps protect the heart from hurt and nurtures and rebuilds the injured heart and personality by supporting and nurturing positive spiritual and soul qualities within the individual These supportive soul qualities are symbolized by the color and fragrance of the bloom, the magnificent expression of the "soul" of the plant.

Among the soul qualities supported are endurance, motivation, resilience, nurture and sustenance.

As one takes the rose flower essence, the personality begins to re-harmonize and balance. It becomes easier to cope with unexpected changes and transitions in life. The following positive spiritual and soul qualities may begin to emerge: appreciation, cherishing, compassion, delight, devotion, endurance, enthusiasm, forgiveness, grace, gratitude, hope, joy, love, optimism, patience, self-generation, self-love, unity.

Of course, it is God's Spirit that ultimately cultivates these spiritual qualities in the human heart. I believe that God has given us rose flower essences to support this process.

For example, *Rosa* **'Double Delight'**, with its large, multi-petaled, bi-colored raspberry/cream blooms and spicy-sweet fragrance, resonates with and supports the spiritual qualities of love, unity and delight. By nurturing the sweetness of self-love through helping to unify the fragmented personality, this rose supports a re-connection with our soul's highest aspirations and expression.

Rosa **'LD Braithwaite'**, a deep red, multi-petaled rose with an exquisite fragrance, supports our life-force energy when we are feeling depleted and "beaten down." This rose essence is regenerative and restorative.

More specific flower essences are similarly described in Chapter Five.

A Unique Interpretation of the Spiritual and Soul Qualities Supported By Rose Flower Essences

Norwegian iridologist and homeopath-homotoxicologist, Ørjan Repaal, has used the rose essences on himself and with clients through my Rose Essence Research Program while it was under the auspices of my former company, Crystal Radiance. He interprets these qualities in a unique way:

> The Rose Essences had a strong and very good energy, and the sensations were distinct and not to be mistaken.

My total impression of these rose essences is, in general, an affecting of the heart, with emotions such as LOVE AND JOY. This is probably the general effect for all the botanical roses.

When dealing with the emotions of love, one needs to know the different sides of this emotion. The English term, 'Love' has a broad meaning. In Greek the word is split up into different words to describe the feeling:

Agape – Love based on PRINCIPLES, like empathy, compassion, self-sacrifice, and so on.
Philia – Love between FRIENDS, like friendship, companionship, and so on.
Storge – Love among FAMILY, like mothers/fathers, love between other family members.
Eros – SEXUAL (romantic) love - by far the best between male and female (when healthy) in a stable relationship.

When using some of the rose flower essences himself and with some of his clients, Repaal found the following associations:

> Rosa **'Double Delight'** – *Philia*
> Rosa **'Evelyn'** – *Storge*
> Rosa **'French Perfume'** – *Eros*
> Rosa **'Guy de Maupassant'** – *Agape, Storge*
> Rosa **'Tiffany'** – *Storge*

These principles closely align with the benefits reported by many essence users and clients whose anecdotal testimonies are offered in following chapters.

Rose flower essences are effective, supportive remedies that help us to make it through tough and painful times. They may also be keys to opening us to sharing love more deeply in our relationships. I am grateful that I have been guided to work with these healing flower remedies because I've witnessed how they've supported so many people through difficult times.

You will find specific healing potentials of 52 roses in Chapter Five, "52 Rose Flower Essences, Their Healing Qualities and Practical Applications."

CHAPTER 3
ROSE FLOWER ESSENCES AND THE
MEMORY OF WATER

The Discovery of "Living Water"

*H*ow can plain old water, into which a flower blossom was once placed and subsequently removed, become a healing flower essence? The secret is that the water is no longer just "plain old water."

Scientific research has brought to light that the very structure of water gives clues to its energetic nature. Water has unique properties making it the perfect carrier of the vibrational healing energies of flowers in the form of flower essences.

The early 20th century researcher, Viktor Schauberger, studied water along with the Earth's natural processes. Schauberger saw water as "living" and based upon his scientific experiments, theorized that water actually has "memory".[1]

Schauberger found that spinning water molecules absorb the frequencies of the chemicals and biological substances that may be surrounding them. He found that water mimics the structure of the microorganisms or chemicals even when they are no longer present. He also found that this structured water even causes the same biological reactions in plants and animals that consume it as the chemicals themselves would have produced.[2]

Since 1994, Japanese researcher, Dr. Masaru Emoto has been offering even more compelling evidence of the phenomenon of water's ability to "remember" and mimic the structure of substances placed into it that are no longer present. Dr. Emoto took hundreds of specimens of water from various sources and conducted creative experiments based upon his belief that water crystals reflect the essence of water. By taking water, freezing it, then examining and photographing the resulting water crystals under a powerful microscope, Dr. Emoto has offered the world visual evidence of Schauberger's theories on the memory of water.

Messages from Water

In his visually stunning books, *The Message from Water, Vol. 1, 2, and 3,* Dr. Emoto shares his groundbreaking research that shows literally dozens of photographs of water, whose structure, or lack thereof, results from its exposure to chemicals, pollution, metal piping, pristine conditions or even music, thoughts, words and substances. What is most amazing and relevant to our discussion is one experiment in particular. The experiment he describes in Volume 1 is titled "Transcribing Aromatherapy Oil Information on Water: Chamomile Water and Fennel Water." Describing the experiment and its results Dr. Emoto says:

> HADO information that aromatherapy oil contains was transcribed* to a water sample and was frozen before taking the crystal's picture. We were surprised to obtain a picture of a crystal that is similar to the look of the flowers that the different aroma oils were made from. These crystals may *resemble the shape of the substance.* (Italics mine).[3]

*Note: It seems that this transcription process involves transmitting the biological information contained in the vial of essential oil to the vial containing water using what appears to be a low frequency electronic amplifier. The particles in the water pick up the electromagnetic information or vibratory pattern from the particles in the essential oil. The vibratory pattern is like a code or signature that healthy water can pick up and transmit. Dr. Emoto is not the first scientist to carry out this type of experiment. In the 1990's French biochemist, Jacques Benvenist, conducted similar experiments, bringing us one step closer to understanding that water retains and transmits information.[4]

The microscopic photographs of the water crystals resulting from Dr. Emoto's experiment are no less than astounding. The frozen crystals of the newly structured water that was exposed through "transcription" (being placed into a vial in proximity to, but not actually touching the vial of water) mimic the actual shape of the chamomile and fennel flowers that made the oils! See photos in his books or on his website: www.hado.net.

This very compelling evidence shows that water, indeed, possesses a type of memory. Charlie Ryrie, an environmental researcher, editor and author of *The Healing Energies of Water* states:

> Healthy water has a strong three-dimensional crystalline microstructure that allows it to collect and transmit information. It is the structure of the water that allows it to communicate…[5]

> To a non-scientist, the idea that water has a memory is not particularly astonishing. Every living thing is affected by its environment, physically and emotionally. Human beings retain impressions of all that happens to us on our journey from life to death…So if we recognize water as a living entity it should be no surprise that it has a memory.[6]

As with flower essences, the most basic principles of the healing science of Homeopathy are based upon this vibrational memory that is displayed by water. By purposely exposing water to subtle energies of plant, animal or mineral substances then diluting and shaking it (succussion),[7] a homeopathic remedy is made. A homeopathic remedy at extreme dilution, still retains the imprint or memory of the original qualities of the substance, even though it no longer contains any measurable molecular evidence of the substance that was originally present.

Homeopathic remedies have been shown to affect the vital force of the physical body on an energetic level. Flower essences, prepared in a similar way (though they may or may not be succussed), likewise affect the human vital force at molecular and sub-molecular energetic levels.

CHAPTER 4
FLOWER ESSENCE HEALING IN YOUR GARDEN

The Garden as a Healing Space

*T*he cure for the stress in your life could literally be lying in your own backyard. Garden environments promote health, inspire tranquility and help to bring balance and a sense of wellbeing. The healing garden beckons, "Come into my peaceful space. Bring me your sorrows, your confusion, your frazzled nerves. Surround yourself with my colors, my freshness and fragrances. Let me be your haven on earth. Leave refreshed and renewed!"

Being out in nature simply makes people feel better. Medical studies have verified the calming benefits of viewing or being in a natural setting:

> "Laboratory and clinical investigations have found that viewing nature settings can produce significant [stress recovery] within less than five minutes, as indicated by positive blood pressure, heart activity, muscle tension and brain electrical activity," concludes Roger S. Ulrich, Ph.D., in a recent summary on the health benefits of gardens.[1]

Programs that utilize horticultural therapy, the use of gardens as rehabilitative settings, have been steadily growing in popularity. Patients recovering from traumatic injury or surgery have shown dramatic improvements in attitude and healing rate when they spend just one hour a day working with the plants or spending time in a therapeutic garden.[2] Restorative garden sanctuaries have also become a hit with stressed-out individuals seeking refuge from the rigors of modern urban life. Whether in a city botanical garden, a community vegetable garden or one's own backyard flower garden, many have found refuge, regeneration and serenity in these garden spaces.

Working with Rose Flower Essences in Your Healing Garden

You can work with the rose flower essences in your healing garden space. By spending time in your garden or in natural outdoor surroundings, you will greatly enhance your therapeutic program with rose flower essences. In the privacy of your garden you can play, dance, ruminate, meditate, sing, journal, dig, water and smell the roses, enjoy the play of light and sound, listen to the buzzing of insects and enjoy the song of birds. While working with your rose flower essences, you may begin to cultivate the qualities of peace, joy, contentment and gratitude in your heart. In the healing garden space you can be alive, spontaneous and child-like, as you work with specific flower essences that nurture these qualities. At the same time you will find yourself less tense and anxious. The outdoors is the perfect place for self-exploration and natural healing.

In the next chapter you will find practical applications on how to enhance your healing while using your rose flower essences in your garden or natural surroundings as healing environments. Feel free to follow these suggestions, modify them, or come up with your own creative ideas.

CHAPTER 5
52 ROSE FLOWER ESSENCES, THEIR HEALING POTENTIALS AND PRACTICAL APPLICATIONS

*T*he following descriptions of the healing potentials of the rose flower essences have evolved over several years of my working closely with them. They have been arrived at through a combination of methods: through experimental research, client work with the essences, prayer and meditation, intuition, oral ingestion, topical application, bath therapy and application via mist spray. I have observed how they have affected me and many clients and users. With more clinical research over the next months and years, these healing potentials will be refined.

Since each person is different from the next, you may be uniquely influenced by these essences. When holding bottles of essences and while using them, I encourage you to quiet yourself, go within and listen to the subtle "voices" of these beautiful flowers. Discover for yourself the wonderful healing gifts their essences may bring to you. As you read the following section, imagine the healing voice of each rose, as if each individual rose is speaking directly to you as it describes itself and its specific healing potentials.

A practical application for each rose essence is included after the description and its healing potentials. In some instances the application is included within the healing potential description.

Please note that the registered 'popular" names of hybrid rose cultivars rarely have anything to do with their soul healing qualities. Some of these names were chosen arbitrarily, or chosen according to the whims of rose hybridizers and enthusiasts for myriad reasons. They are named after movie stars and personalities: 'Elizabeth Taylor', 'Whoopi Goldberg', 'Betty Boop'; authors: 'Guy de Maupassant'; famous rose gardeners or hybridizers: 'Gertrude Jekyll', 'Jayne Austin'; and even cars: 'Chrysler Imperial'. Though many of these names are clever, cute or catchy, I encourage you to relate to each rose and its essence as you would naturally: by its beauty, color, fragrance and healing potentials.

'Altissimo'

I am a deep, velvety red climbing rose. My large, clustered blooms have seven petals. I am mildly fragrant. I bloom repeatedly during my growing season and can reach up to 10 feet in height. My foliage is deep green.

Healing potentials: I assist your body to self-heal and to better endure stress.

Application: Apply to the base of the spine and to the heart area and crown of the head. Use the single rose essence to deepen spiritual contemplation. Sit near the rose in a garden. Sense the life-force of the plant, as you work with its flower essence.

'Anastasia'

I am a hybrid tea rose with a medium-sized double bloom. My 30 petals are a lovely white blend and I love to bloom repeatedly throughout the season. My foliage is a dark green. Though my life-force is vigorous, my fragrance is light and airy.

Healing potentials: I help you to embody your pure child-like innocence and adaptability.

> *Application: Take this essence when the need to adapt to new and unexpected situations arises. Affirm and nurture yourself by taking this essence while in a garden of roses and other beautiful flowers. Sing, dance, play, create in the garden, alone or with a partner or group. Let go and enjoy yourself!*

'Arizona'

I am a grandiflora rose with double medium-sized yellow-orange blooms. I love to bloom repeatedly throughout the season to bring my strong, pleasant fragrance to all who walk by. My leaves are dark, shiny green and leathery. My life-force is strong and vital.

Healing potentials: I help you to strengthen your emotional connections with others. I support your central nervous system as you adjust to these new patterns of being.

> *Application: Use this essence when doing deep, conscious emotional work with the clear intention to open to love. Apply topically to the heart area. May be used as a support when undergoing spiritual counseling for emotional cleansing.*

'Bill Warriner'

I am a pink floribunda rose. My bloom is coral pink or salmon pink with 20–25 petals. My light fragrance graces the wind throughout my long growing season. I have dark green leaves that shine in the sun.

Healing potentials: I am the rose for you who over-works, frets and worries. I help you find a calm and tranquil heartbeat and rhythm of breath that slows down frantic thought processes. I help to bring you back to equilibrium and to find reverie and sanctuary.

Application: Take this essence when in need of comfort and share with others who need comforting. Use when feeling "pulled apart" by doing too many things at once and when feeling bombarded by excessive internal or external stimuli. Take while in a natural setting and slowly and rhythmically breathe in the stillness and freshness of nature's sanctuary.

'Bonica'

I am a shrub rose. My double blooms are medium pink, fading to light pink at the edges and are 40 petals full. I have small, dark green semi-glossy leaves. I have very little fragrance.

Healing potentials: Where there is turmoil, I offer you a sense of peace.

Application: Use orally when feeling stressed by inner conflict or by conflict with another. Take the essence to help resolve turmoil within a group that is working together. It is helpful when all parties take the essence. May also be mist sprayed in the room or environment.

'Brandy'

I am a beautiful hybrid tea rose with coral to apricot double blooms that are 4 inches wide with 25–30 delicate petals. My sweet, fruity fragrance is strong, to attract the curious nose. I am abundant with medium green, glossy leaves. I am hardy, blooming repeatedly throughout my growing season. I like the afternoon shade.

Healing potentials: Meditate upon my bloom and fragrance and use my essence to assist you as you envision your greatest God-given creative potential.

Application: Meditate upon this rose in the garden and take its essence orally as you contemplate your spiritual path and goals. Consciously take in its fragrance and periodically gaze into the lovely bloom to receive subtle inspiration. Ask for guidance from God and angels. The best time to do this is in the freshness of early morning, immediately after sunrise.

'Brass Band'

I am a floribunda rose. My large, ruffled blooms of 25–30 petals are a lovely warm blend of apricot and melon-pink with subtle golden apricot reverses. I love to bloom heavily, provided the desert weather is cool. My bush is full of medium sized green leaves and I offer you a fragrance just detectable on the cool breeze.

Healing potentials: I inspire you to seek fulfillment in your life. I help you to realize that you are so very much loved. Hear angelic symphonies in celebration.

Application: Take this essence orally or apply to heart area and crown of the head. Sing songs of celebration to God's creation.

'Bride'

I am a pink hybrid tea shrub rose with large, 4-inch blooms with a high center. My blooms scroll open gracefully and my fragrance is fairly strong but not as sweet as the red roses. I like to bloom repeatedly during the season of warm weather and bright sun.

Healing potentials: I support you to discover gratitude and love for simple and beautiful things. I am an essence for those who wish to simplify their lives and who also wish to connect more with nature.

Application: Take this essence orally. Place a few drops on the heart area, brow and crown of the head. Then vow to eliminate the things that clutter your life. Take also when camping and hiking to gain new outlooks in nature.

'Camara'

I am a brilliant vermillion red hybrid tea rose. My large, 4-inch bloom has a light fragrance. My large leaves are a medium to dark green.

Healing potentials: I support you as you breathe in the radiance of joy. I center you and calm your inner stirrings of doubt, fostering a sense of confidence.

Application: Apply this essence at the base of the spine, heart area and take orally. It can be very supportive during those uncertain years of adolescence or when revisiting one's "emotional adolescence".

'Cherish'

I am a floribunda rose, with a hybrid tea form. My coral pink double blooms have 26–28 petals and grow among my dark, green leaves. You will detect a mild fragrance among my 3-4 foot tall canes.

Healing potentials: I encourage you to cherish things dear. I support your heart's sharing of love.

Application: Take orally, apply to the heart, the base of the skull (medulla oblongata), and the inside of the wrists. Close your eyes and clearly visualize people, animals, places that you cherish. Then, place them into your heart.

'Chrysler Imperial'

I am a hybrid tea rose with deep red, double 4-inch blooms. My foliage is a deep green and is semi-glossy. I am extremely fragrant.

Healing potentials: I support the meridians that energize your five senses through your central nervous system.

Application: Apply this essence to the heart area, back of the wrists, behind the knee and at the base of the spine. Place a full dropper in a warm bath and soak with the petals of this rose floating all around you. Enjoy with all of your senses!

'Crystalline'

I am a pristine white hybrid tea rose with double blooms of 30–35 petals. My leaves are dark green. I carry no fragrance in my many blossoms among my 3–4 foot canes.

Healing potentials: I promote loving harmony and endurance in your relationships and a deeper spiritual journey.

Application: Spray this essence within the living or work space that you share. Place a vase of freshly cut blooms and a bowl of spring water containing a fully opened floating bloom of this rose as a centerpiece where prayer and meals are shared.

'Double Delight'

I am a hybrid tea bush or climber. I have raspberry and cream dual-colored blooms with 30–35 petals. My blooms are double and I have medium dark green foliage. I love warm days and cool nights. The desert spring and late fall seasons are my favorite. I have a very spicy-sweet fragrance. I am a popular rose due to my color, form and fragrance.

Healing potentials: I encourage a desire for unity, delight and aspiration for true love within the heart and soul.

Application: Take orally and apply to the inner wrists and heart area as well as on the calf below the knee. Groups that aspire to unify in values and goals through heart-felt cooperation will greatly benefit when using this essence together orally or by mist spray.

'Eglantine'

I am an English shrub rose with large double, cupped, medium-pink blooms. I am quite fragrant and bushy.

Healing potentials: I help to align and balance your bio-energy field. I promote a greater sense of health and wellbeing.

Application: Apply this essence to the soles of your feet, palms, heart area and crown. Mist spray around the body, while breathing deeply.

'Electron'

I am a stunning hybrid tea rose. My double blossoms are up to 5 inches wide and are electric pink in color, blooming all season long. My life-force and fragrance are strong and I have many thorns and medium green, leathery leaves.

Healing potentials: I help you to attune to body and earth rhythms. This occurs within the fluids of your spine, nervous system and cells.

Application: Take orally and apply behind ears, to the heart area and at the base of the spine. Sit quietly in a secluded natural space. Listen to your heartbeat and to the sounds in your surroundings as far away as possible. The therapist and client may use this essence during Cranial-Sacral Therapy to enhance sensitivity to cranial and spinal fluid rhythms.

'Elizabeth Taylor'

I am an elegantly dark pink hybrid tea rose with lovely double blooms of 30–35 petals that are deeper pink on the edges. My leaves are deep green. I will captivate you with my spicy fragrance in the warmest of weather, which is my favorite.

Healing potentials: I support you as you center yourself, through walking and moving meditation and contemplation.

Application: Take orally, apply to the base of spine, sacrum, heart and crown of the head. Use with walking prayers through natural outdoor formations.

'Evelyn'

I am an Old Garden-English shrub rose. My lovely double apricot pink blossoms appear as rosettes and have over 45 petals! They are 3–4 inches wide. I like to bloom repeatedly throughout my growing season to thrill all those who see me. In addition, I gift everyone within the area with my immense, lovely sweet fragrance.

Healing potentials: I inspire you to love deeply, to contemplate your destiny of service on Earth. I encourage peaceful cooperation.

Application: Take this essence orally and place a few drops on the heart, sacrum, solar plexus and crown of head. Sit upon the earth in a lovely garden or natural space and envision a growing, expanding light and energy of trust and cooperation among yourself and the flowers, plants trees, creatures and people of God's earth.

'Fair Bianca'

I am an English shrub rose. My pristine white blooms are double, 3 inches wide with a green center, growing on 3-foot high canes. My bright green foliage catches the eye as my extremely fragrant blooms repeat throughout the year. I am a David Austin rose, introduced in 1982.

Healing potentials: I bring love-song and beauty to the heart. I help to nurture your heart-song. I am an essence for the singer.

Application: Use this essence in conjunction with singing and birdsong. Apply this essence to the heart center and crown of head. While in a backyard, garden or park, remain very quiet and listen for the most beautiful birdsong you can hear. Take the essence once your ears settle upon this lovely song. Close your eyes and allow the song's beauty to enter your ears and heart, giving thanks for this divine gift. Take this essence while cultivating your own singing voice.

'Fragrant Plum'

Purple is my coloring. I am a cool lavender hybrid tea rose. My blooms are edged with an even deeper purple and are richly fragrant, showing the classic hybrid tea form. I am extremely hardy with large, rich green, glossy leaves.

Healing potentials: I help you to become aware of more subtle energies, encouraging stillness, a quieting, and healing.

Application: Apply a few drops to the base of spine, heart, throat and brow. Also, place a drop in the center of each palm to become aware of subtle bio-energies.

'French Perfume'

I am a hybrid tea rose with a classic rose fragrance, while my petals are a light cream color with a raspberry edge.

Healing potentials: I inspire you to know yourself, as a spirit walking, clothed in God's light, perfumed in the fragrance of roses. I inspire contentment.

Application: Take orally and apply to solar plexus, heart and crown. Then praise, pray and "light bathe" in God's glorious presence.

'Gertrude Jekyll'

I am an Old Garden–English shrub rose. My blossoms are deep pink and are 4 inches wide. I stun the eye with my 45 petals that curl and curve within the rosette of the bloom. I bloom several times during my growing season, just in case you missed me the first time.

Healing potentials: I encourage you to become aligned to God's higher purpose for you. I help you to honor yourself.

Application: Take orally and apply to the base of the spine, heart and crown. Use while contemplating your life's unique higher purpose.

'Granada'

I am a hybrid tea rose that blooms abundantly all season long. My blooms are 4–5 inches wide and are a pleasant blend of light orange, pink and light yellow. They are double with 18–25 petals with a spicy, sweet fragrance that will entice you. I am a prolific bloomer.

Healing potentials: I help you to maintain focus as you move through changes and transitions in your life.

Application: Take this essence orally and apply to sacrum, solar plexus, heart and brow. Also, mist spray around the body. Do deep breathing to help you to de-stress and balance your nervous system.

'Grand Impression'

I am a hybrid tea rose with very large, double blooms that are a salmon yellow with apricot yellow reverses. I grow in small clusters among my large, semi-glossy dark green leaves and lightly thorny stems. I offer you a sweet fragrance. I love to repeat my blossoming all season long for your pleasure.

Healing potentials: I bring you zip and zing, zow and wow! I energize and revitalize, preparing you for physical activity and exercise. I promote endurance.

Application: Take orally and/or apply to the base of the spine and heart and crown. Take essence 5–15 minutes before doing prolonged stretching, deep breathing or any moderate physical exercise.

'Guy de Maupassant'

I am a floribunda-romantica rose. My large, double blooms are medium pink and bloom in small clusters. I am very fragrant with a scent similar to apples. I love to repeat my blooms throughout the growing season. My leaves are large and shiny, dark green. I am a rose that was introduced in France.

Healing potentials: I help you to become more empathic. I support understanding and forgiveness within your heart. I encourage you to consciously choose to be compassionate.

Application: Take orally and apply to the root area, heart area and crown area.

'Harlequin'

I am a hybrid tea rose. My double blooms are lavender and mauve blend with white reverses and are 30 petals full. I give you a pleasant, sweet fragrance as you lean in to smell my flowers among my medium-sized, dark green-gray leaves.

Healing potentials: I support your efforts to see and understand the pattern of Love (Christ) that underlies and permeates all matter. I help you see through the heart, clearly.

Application: Take this essence orally and apply to heart, brow and crown centers. Use when you wish to "see" and feel beyond the surface appearance of things in order to experience a sense of the "divine moment".

31

'Jayne Austin'

I am an Old Garden-English shrub rose. My 3-inch peach-apricot blooms are shaped like full rosettes. They have a honey-colored center and carry a surprising pepper-like fragrance. My foliage is a glossy dark green. My life-force is strong and vigorous.

Healing potentials: I harmonize your heart with your art. I assist the artist within to manifest herself. I support you to flow with the cascade of creative energies that fuel your artistic endeavors.

Application: Take orally and apply this to the sacrum, solar plexus, heart and throat areas. Use this essence when beginning any creative or artistic activity, especially where improvisation is involved.

'Just Joey'

I am a stunning hybrid tea rose perpetual with plenty of soft orange-apricot double blooms. My 25–30 petals are serrated on the edges. This gives me a unique look, setting me apart from typical hybrid tea roses. My fragrance is strong and fruity. I have dark, glossy leaves and I love hot weather and a lot of sun.

Healing potentials: I am a guardian rose. My purpose is to bring a sense of support and love during times of extreme stress and duress. Within this sense of protection, your child-self senses her true state of innocence, joy and wonder.

Application: Take orally or apply to the sacrum, solar plexus and heart areas when undergoing stresses that trigger a regression to a child-like neediness. This essence can emotionally support when one is convalescing from a physical illness.

'LD Braithwaite'

I am an Old Garden-English shrub rose. My full, double cupped blooms are a beautiful burgundy red. I can be a huge bush, up to 5 feet tall and 7 feet wide! My foliage is healthy and green with a bit of a gloss. I love to grow vigorously throughout my growing season and produce abundant blooms for your viewing pleasure.

Healing potentials: I catalyze your self-generation, energizing your nervous system.

Application: Take orally and apply to the root, sacrum and heart areas, base of the neck (medulla oblongata) and crown.

'Lanvin'

I am a yellow hybrid tea rose with contrasting reddish-green foliage.

Healing potentials: I inspire you to remember that God is the One who mends, and that, when all seems lost, you will have the courage you need to carry on.

Application: Take orally or apply to the sacrum, solar plexus and heart centers. Use for support with joyful energies when you find yourself descending into sadness or despair.

'Louise Odier'

I am an Old Garden-Bourbon rose. My very fragrant full double blooms are medium pink and I compact 35 40 petals within a 3-inch width. I have a classic "old garden rose" form. My foliage is light to medium green and I have a few surprise thorns, so be careful when handling. I bloom abundantly when the season is at mid-point.

Healing potentials: I bring out the optimism in your heart. Dancing is how I manifest my energies in your body, so take my essence and dance beautifully.

Application: Take orally and apply to the root, heart and crown areas, as well as to the wrists. Then dance, dance, dance!

'Madame Isaac Pereire'

I am an Old English-Garden rose—a bourbon. My color is deep pink with red to purple shading. My blooms are double and large, 3–4 inches, and I have thorny canes with semi-glossy green leaves. I am intensely fragrant with a sweet, rosy aroma. I am a huge, abundantly flowering shrub, 14–16 feet across.

Healing potentials: I inspire an awareness of deep love and gratitude.

Application: Take orally and apply topically to heart and crown. Then give thanks for all of your gifts.

'Melody Parfumee'

I am a grandiflora rose with beautiful double purple blooms with a lighter silvery plum reverse. I have a sweet to spicy Damask fragrance that caresses your senses as I bloom throughout the season. My leaves are medium-sized and a shiny green.

Healing potentials: Clarity is my domain. I help you to find moments of crystalline light and clarity.

Application: Take orally and apply to the base of the spine, heart, throat, brow and crown when preparing to meditate upon or contemplate a topic.

34

'Mister Lincoln'

I am a deep red hybrid tea rose. My petals are like velvet to the touch, all 30–35 of them, in my large, double bloom. I am famous for my enveloping fragrance, so I am very popular as a cut flower. My leaves are a vigorous deep green color.

Healing potentials: I am a rose of profound grounding when you are feeling spacey.

Application: Take orally and apply to base of spine, soles of feet, heart and wrists. Sit in stillness, close your eyes and breathe deeply to feel more grounded.

'Mon Cheri'

I am a deep pink hybrid tea rose with large 4-inch blooms that give off a light fragrance that will grace your senses. I like to change colors, starting off as bright pink with red edges, slowly deepening to red with the light of the sun. My stems are thorny and my leaves are dark green and glossy.

Healing potentials: With prayer, I support perceiving and experiencing the spiritual dimensions. I help you heighten your awareness and experience of love as true and enduring.

Application: Take orally and apply this essence to the root, heart, brow and crown areas.

'Pat Austin'

I am an Old Garden-English shrub rose. My large, double blooms are deeply cupped and display two tones of copper coloring with bright copper inside and yellow-orange on the outside. I offer a classic, sweet tea-like fragrance to the discerning nose. I bloom in spurts during my growing season. My leaves are a medium to dark green.

Healing potentials: I foster your enthusiasm for spiritual growth and physical healing. I inspire you to create healing environments in nature (contemplation gardens, prayer sanctuaries, etc.)

Application: Take orally and apply to sacral, solar plexus, heart and crown areas. Apply also to the palms and soles of feet. Use with the intention to create a healing and inspirational space in nature.

'Paul Shirville'

I am a very fragrant hybrid tea rose with high-centered double, salmon-pink blooms that repeat throughout the season. My leaves are large and semi-glossy dark green, providing a complementary background for my abundant pink blossoms.

Healing potentials: I attune your ear to celestial symphonies and healing sounds, subtle harmonies and rhythms in earth and sea. I help the musician and composer bring forth music whose sources are subtle realms of sound and light.

Application: Apply to root, heart, brow and crown areas. Apply a drop also behind each ear. Close your eyes and open your hearing to the lapping waves of the sea, lake, or the sounds in a quiet garden or woods. Allow your inner musician to be inspired deeply and lovingly by the heart of nature.

36

'Perdita'

I am an English shrub rose. My blossoms are an apricot blend, have 40 petals and they grow in clusters. I bloom repeatedly throughout the growing season. At times a light scent can be detected among my glossy green leaves.

Healing potentials: I am a connector of nerve impulses along your spine. I nurture energy to your heart, amplifying a sense of hope, faith and charity.

Application: Take orally and put a few drops into a warm bath. Submerge yourself and relax as you contemplate how you may creatively embody hope, faith and charity in your life. May also be added to massage oil for a healing back massage.

'Pristine'

I am a hybrid tea rose with white blossoms tinged with a pink blush. My fragrance is light. I am a popular wedding or anniversary rose, symbolic of the pristine bride on her wedding day.

Healing potentials: I bring to you the gift of calm and serenity as I help to balance your thoughts and calm your heart. I can foster a heightened sensory perception and deeper spiritual insight as I help to balance your nervous system.

Application: Apply this essence to the base of the spine, base of the neck, heart and brow areas. Mist spray around head with eyes closed.

'Regatta'

I am a hybrid tea perpetual rose. My 35-petaled double blooms are a beautiful peachy pink reminiscent of the dawn. I offer a lovely raspberry-like fragrance. I like to branch out and I am quite bushy.

Healing potentials: I bring sweetness and balance to the realm of your experiences and self-expressions. I assist you in harmonizing your creative endeavors with your soul's aspirations.

Application: Apply to the palms of the hands, root, heart, and throat and crown areas. Use when embarking upon any newly inspired creative activity.

'Royal Dane'

I am a hybrid tea rose also known as 'Troika'. My double blooms are a beautiful blend of pink and copper-orange with 30 petals. I have a sweet delicate fragrance. I love to bloom several times during the growing season. My foliage is medium green and shiny. I hold up well in the desert climate.

Healing potentials: I set the stage for catching various aromas through your sense of smell. I am the quintessential rose essence for aromatherapists and those who must discern subtle differences between scents. You may also take my essence as you prepare your meals and before dining, for greater culinary enjoyment.

Application: Take orally and apply to sacrum, solar plexus, heart, brow and crown areas.

'Royal Wedding'

I am a floribunda rose with very large, full, double blooms that are blended pink and yellow. My blooms have 60 very fragrant petals. My leaves are medium-sized and a semi-glossy dark green in color. As I am a repeat bloomer, people love to cut my blooms for vases.

Healing potentials: I assist in bringing forth the qualities of sincere adoration and spiritual devotion.

Application: Take orally and apply to the solar plexus, heart and crown areas. Focus yourself and set the intention within your heart during personal times of prayer and devotion.

'Sea Pearl'

I am known as both a floribunda and a hybrid tea rose. My elegant blooms are double and 4 ½ inches in size. They have 24 light- to medium-pink petals with cream-yellow reverses. My long stems have many thorns among my dark green foliage. I am hardy in the warm weather, but my fragrance is very light so you'll find it only when I first bloom.

Healing potentials: I help you to appreciate all of you, to accept assets and liabilities. I nurture your heart and encourage adaptability, perseverance and resilience.

Application: Take orally and apply to the solar plexus, heart, crown, and to the base of the neck. Use when in doubt about your abilities and when feeling discouraged.

'Summer Fashion'

I am a gorgeous floribunda rose. My double bloom is colored yellow-pink with 30 elegantly ruffled petals. I like to bloom repeatedly during my growing season to offer you my wonderfully fruity fragrance. My leaves are large and semi-glossy. People love to cut and display my flowers.

Healing potentials: I stimulate your senses to open and to take in the earth's abundant beauty.

Application: Take orally and apply this essence to the solar plexus, heart and crown areas. Use when out in a garden, park, forest, to enhance awareness and the enjoyment of your nurturing surroundings.

'Summer's Kiss'

I am hybrid tea rose with many names. I am also known as 'Meinivoz', 'Moondance', 'Paul Ricard', and 'Spirit of Peace'. My large, double blooms are a cream-yellow blend and offer a light, pleasant fragrance.

Healing potentials: I inspire you to move fluidly from inspiration to trust and self-confidence through contentment, joy and laughter. I assist you in becoming more fully and playfully human.

Application: Take orally and apply to solar plexus, heart and crown areas. Mist spray in your environment. Then laugh and play!

'Sunset Celebration'

I am a beautiful hybrid tea shrub rose. My bloom is an apricot-amber blend. My fragrance is fruity.

Healing potentials: I inspire you to use your heart-inspired talents to uplift others. I am the rose for the caregiver who wishes to offer heartfelt support to others.

Application: Take orally and apply to the sacrum, heart, and crown. Take this essence while gazing at the night sky, and enjoy the healing energies and inspirations of starlight.

'Tamora'

I am an old garden shrub rose. My medium-sized cupped blooms are a lovely apricot-yellow with 40 petals that are quite fragrant. My leaves are small and dark green.

Healing potentials: I am a rose for the seeker and the inventor. I urge on the curious child-heart that explores under rocks, in ponds and streams. I bring forth the awe, adventure, play and discovery that fuel the activity of invention.

Application: Take orally and apply to sacrum, solar plexus, and crown areas. Apply also to the palms of the hands.

'Tiffany'

I am a hybrid tea rose with a pink-yellow blend and double 4–5 inch blossoms of 25–30 petals with a high center and a yellow base. I am quite bushy, with many dark green stems and leaves. I love hot summers, when you can experience my strong, fruity fragrance. I am one of the most popular hybrid tea roses. I also grow as a climbing rose.

Healing potentials: I bring you the possibility of love and enjoyment of the moment. I warm your heart's tenderness. I support and encourage you to love yourself and to make this self-love an offering of service to the world.

Application: Take orally and apply to solar plexus, heart and crown areas.

'Timeless'

I am a lightly fragrant, red hybrid tea rose. My double blooms are quite elegant, 4 inches wide, with 25–30 petals that bloom in clusters. My stems are long and shiny and my leaves are a glossy dark green.

Healing potentials: I deepen your heart-connection with nature and earth. I also help to foster sincerity in human relationships.

Application: Apply this essence to the root, and crown areas. Sit and contemplate the earth's beauty and the beauty in others. Sit under a tree and write in your journal about your musings.

'Tineke'

I am a hybrid tea rose with resplendently colored medium-large pearly white blooms with a hint of green. My dark green stems have only a few thorns and my leaves are also dark green. I am one of the most popular white hybrid tea roses.

Healing potentials: I offer you a glimpse of true love and the knowing that you are a priceless pearl, more valuable than diamonds. I help you to share love's purity.

Application: Take orally and apply the heart and crown areas.

'Touch of Class'

I am a hybrid tea rose with a double 4–5 inch blossom of 33 petals with a mild fragrance. My color ranges from medium pink to a shading of coral and orange. My foliage is dark green and semi-glossy.

Healing potentials: Joy, Joy, Joy! This is my offering to you! I bring dolphin-like spontaneity, opening potentials for spiritual growth.

Application: Take orally and apply to the root, sacral, solar plexus, heart and crown areas.

'Tournament of Roses'

I am a grandiflora rose with a light coral bloom with deep pink-coral reverses. My blooms are 3–4 inches wide with 25–40 delicate petals that have only the slightest fragrance. My foliage is semi-glossy dark green.

Healing potentials: I energize your bio-energy system. I encourage balance and alignment within your creativity. With my essence, you may create beautiful forms.

Application: Take orally and apply to sacrum, heart and crown centers and mist spray around the body.

'Y'ves Piaget'

I am a fuchsia pink hybrid tea rose. My stems and leaves are medium to dark green. My double blooms can be a huge 5 inches in diameter with 40 petals! It's no surprise, then, that I have a very strong fragrance.

Healing potentials: I inspire patience, bringing gladness and joy to your heart.

Application: Take this essence orally and apply to the root, heart and crown areas. Nurture yourself and be patient as you release old hurts in order to open and receive abundant joy.

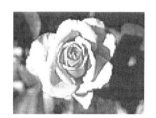

CHAPTER 6
13 COMBINATION FORMULAS

W hile working with the roses and other flowers together, I've found that they so beautifully complement one another in synergistic formulas. I also began to hear beautiful messages in my meditations and contemplations as I used the essences. I wrote them down over a period of months and then confirmed them over the years. These lovely, nurturing meditations preface the description of each combination formula of rose and other flower essences below.

Each combination formula contains a rose variety* to assist in the healing and expansion of the heart. Other flowers work synergistically with the rose in the formula to complement, focus, attune and amplify the healing qualities of the formulas. Case stories are included with several of the formulas in order to show how these formulas have benefited others. The names have been changed in the interest of privacy.

* Rose flower varieties are indicated by the word *Rosa* followed by the name in quotation marks. The healing qualities of the other flowers have been thoroughly documented and are referred to in Appendix C.

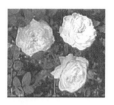

Surround yourself with Love's compassion.
Give yourself a rose.
Forgive yourself and
all who may have hurt your heart.

Compassion ~ Forgiveness
Rosa 'Guy de Maupassant'
Beech and Lilac Flowers

*T*his essence fosters compassion and forgiveness as one continually surrenders to love.

Many of us tend to get caught up in the hustle and bustle of modern society. We rush from here to there, eat fast food and wind up on the wheel of "doing-ness." There is nothing wrong with "doing." The laundry has to get done and that report due on the boss's desk helps keep the company running smoothly. But, in our rush of doing, we lose touch with *being.*

In *being,* we begin to find compassion for ourselves and for others. In this space we once again ground into our body, hear our heartbeat, feel the rise and fall of our breath.

This essence formula contains the pink rose, *'Guy de Maupassant'.* This rose has 90-100 petals, and its pink color represents sympathy and compassion. Thus, we can feel for others deeply and learn to forgive each person, as well as ourselves, as many times as this rose has petals. After forgiving one hundred times, forgiveness becomes a natural part of our being. As Christ demonstrated, forgiveness must be a constant state of the heart.[1]

Beech flower encourages compassion and a relaxing of strict, inflexible attitudes towards others, while lilac flower assists one in the process of forgiving.

Pattern of Imbalance: Resentment projected towards others and God, unforgiving attitude.

Affirmation
**I fully and unconditionally forgive myself
and others who have harmed me.
I am radiant with compassion.**

KEYWORDS
unforgiving of self and others ~ Forgiving
self-will ~ Surrender
doing ~ Being
hardness of heart ~ Compassionate

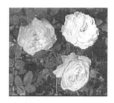

Gratitude evaporates clouds' heaviness.
Sun's light is revealed once more.

Faith in the Storm
Rosa 'Crystalline'
Morning Glory and Self-Heal Flowers

*T*he beauty of the colors in a rainbow during a downpour is a sign of hope. Likewise, a rainbow's colors remind us to be hopeful and to trust in God in the midst of storm and tears. With this essence, one is reminded that just as the rainbow is created by the light of the sun as well as the raindrops, God's light continues to shine in the midst of our inner storms, offering insight and comfort.

'Crystalline' rose, with its pristine white bloom, holds the promise of healing coming from a deeper spiritual reality. Its strong stem and dark green foliage bring hardiness and the strength to endure and ride out the storm.

Morning Glory flower helps us to break away from destructive, addictive habits and find spiritual renewal, while Self-Heal flower encourages us to have faith in the healing process.

Pattern of Imbalance: Loss of faith, hopeless, despairing.

Affirmation
I have faith in God. I have faith in the healing process.

<u>KEYWORDS</u>
despairing ~ Faithful
floundering ~ Enduring
hopeless ~ Hopeful

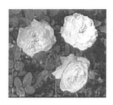

*Have compassion for yourself on the day
the clouds are overcast in the sky of your heart.
Remember, there is always a seed of hope lying inside of
you. Nurture it. Water it.
Even with your own tears.*

Grief Relief
Rosa 'Y'ves Piaget'
Rosa 'Double Delight'
Ocotillo Flower

Grieving is a natural part of the healing process when we have suffered a loss. Without grief, we would not be able to let go, move on, evolve and grow. This essence supports the initial stages of grief, as it waxes and wanes, comes and goes in waves.

The mauve-pink energies of *'Y'ves Piaget'* rose support us to be patient and tender with ourselves, and that the shedding of tears is part of the cleansing process.

'Double Delight' rose, with its lovely bi-color petals (white, with pink edges that deepen in sunlight), helps the heart hold its promise of unity and the aspiration for spiritual love.

Ocotillo is a desert cactus-flower that reminds us to have faith during the time we are in the desert of grief and supports our ability to accept our losses during the grieving process.

Pattern of Imbalance: Unable to let go of grudges, resentment, feelings of abandonment due to loss, living in the past.

Affirmation
**I let go of all past sufferings.
I embrace joy and wholeness in the present.**

<u>KEYWORDS</u>
grief ~ Joy
loss ~ Faith
holding onto loss ~ Accepting Loss and Moving On

Sharon's Story: From Grief to Excitement

Sharon had just separated from her husband who had moved out of the house. Though she felt positive about their decision to separate, she found herself feeling very lonely at times and longing to go back with him again, even though it was against her better judgment.

Sharon started to take *Grief Relief* essence to help her to accept her loss and to encourage her to move on without him. She took the essence under her tongue in the morning and at night, finding that also adding it to her bath supported her in a surprising way. As she lay in the tub, she'd breathe deeply and think about her loneliness. Eventually, she would weep and verbalize her feelings as she became aware of them.

After this happened on several occasions, Sharon even began to expect it. Her grief eased and she was able to begin planting the seeds of starting her own business, a goal she had put off during the relationship. She felt less burdened emotionally and even felt excitement about her business venture, now having more energy to devote to it.

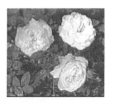

Move towards a oneness within yourself ~
As the rose plant channels all of its energy towards the
pinnacle of its expression ~
the beautiful blossom.
So too, that blossom, which symbolizes your heart, is the
expression of whom you are in God's heart.

Heart Balance
Rosa 'Timeless'
Rosemary and Sweet White Violet Flowers

*T*o gaze into a rose blossom is to be fully transported into the present moment where time stands still and no longer seems to exist. On the other hand, to feel the debilitating emotions that cause us to be skeptical, cynical or distrustful keeps us stuck in the past, unable to break free of the wheel of pain and time, so to speak. We become self-protecting, selfish and self-focused.

The rose, *'Timeless'*, with it's deep red vibration, helps to ground us and balance our body's energies. It helps us to center in our heart and inspires us towards self-love, which we then can allow to blossom and open to trust and share with others.

Rosemary flower strengthens the heart and our ability to trust ourselves.

Sweet White Violet flower encourages us to be open and to nurture trust in our interactions.

Pattern of Imbalance: Hardness of heart, distrust, skepticism, cynicism, inability to share sincerely.

Affirmation
My heart is now flowering in fullness and trust in God's Loving Light.

KEYWORDS
self-protective ~Trusting
skeptical ~ Certain
selfish ~ Sharing

Aida's Story: From Isolation to Trust

Aida found it hard to trust anyone. If you wanted her trust, you had to earn it, and even then she was always waiting for the other shoe to drop. She had trouble communicating openly with her friends. They always described her as being "stoic". Suspecting that it was a heart issue, she was drawn to the rose flower essence formulas. She took *Heart Balance* formula twice a day for 4 weeks.

During that time Aida began to become aware of buried feelings and fear of abandonment she felt concerning her mother as she was growing up. She realized that this played into her reluctance to trust others in her relationships, especially with women. She also realized that this was why she'd always formed relationships with *nurturing* men.

Her awareness was heightened by a physical release of old stomach and abdominal pains, which eventually eased as she processed her feelings. A few weeks later, Aida began to reconnect with female friends she had isolated from for several years. She found herself calling them on the telephone more often, sharing her feelings and spending time with them. As she reconnected, she found herself willing to trust her friends and share more openly with them.

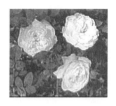

Listen to your heart.
Connect the heart-mind circuit.
A child laughs.
It is your soul's musing.

Lightness of Heart
Rosa 'Anastasia'
Zinnia Flower

*T*his essence formula relieves stress in the mental body, bringing spiritual energies to intellectual activities. It helps to take attention out of the head and brings it more into the emotional energy centers, especially the heart, alleviating a "too serious" attitude.

Are you the type of person who takes everything too seriously? You have trouble enjoying anything, especially with other people. You find it hard to let go, let down your guard, be spontaneous and have fun. You don't have a clue what activities would be fun for you and can't even remember the last time you did anything with the reckless abandon that you experienced as a child. This essence to the rescue!

'Anastasia' rose helps us to embody the child-like spirit. It's clear, pristine white blossom is exceptionally beautiful, like the pure, innocence of a child. It is a hardy rose that's easy to cultivate and adapts well. Children have remarkable adaptability and we all know how "hardy" they can be, (to the point of exhaustion for adults).

Zinnia flower encourages connection with the playful, joyful child-self within each of us.

Pattern of Imbalance: Over-worry, overly intellectual and serious, unable to play.

Affirmation
**I let go of the heaviness of all distracting thoughts.
I allow myself to have fun.**

KEYWORDS
worrisome ~ Joyful
self-conscious ~ Spontaneous
distracted ~ Focused
serious ~ Playful

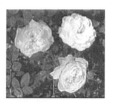

Openly accept love and express love.
This is the beginning of true freedom.

Love's Expression
Rosa 'Sea Pearl'
Daffodil Flower

This formula helps the heart to mature and flower, encouraging a radiant expression of love as emotions find equilibrium and balance.

Once you begin to live in a space of unconditional love for self and others, you begin to express that love.

The "foundation " of this essence is the rose 'Sea Pearl', a lovely cream yellow-pink rose that helps to balance chaotic emotions as it balances the heart and inspires affection and appreciation for self and others.

Daffodil flower encourages self-esteem and acceptance.

Pattern of Imbalance: Unable to express love verbally, physically, emotionally, defensive, aggressive, arrogant.

Affirmation
I express love unconditionally. I give and receive love graciously.

<u>KEYWORDS</u>
aggressive ~ Expressive of Love
arrogant ~ Appreciative
defensive ~ Understanding

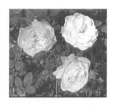

Love is the driving force.
It is the same force that drives the beating of your heart,
the beading of the silvery dew, the blossoming of the rose.

Love Source
Rosa 'Madame Isaac Pereire'
Echinacea and Primrose Flowers

*I*nspiring one to find and strengthen one's connection with God's wellspring where love resides, this formula encourages a desire for heart-connection with the Infinite Source.

When we are disconnected from God, The Source, we are out of balance with all things and thrown way off center. Lack of a spiritual connection can make us literally feel "dried up". Our vital life-force diminishes and we suffer without much hope of permanent reprieve.

Echinacea flower helps to restore our vital energy.

Primrose flower symbolizes the divine spark within the heart. It supports *'Madame Isaac Pereire'* rose, whose deep pink vibration grounds us in deep gratitude and thankfulness as we remember that all in life is a gift from God and that we can grow and learn in all situations.

Pattern of Imbalance: Inability to pray or meditate with focus, feeling disconnected, alienated or separated from God.

Affirmation
I find strength within the heart of God.
I share with the love in my heart.

<u>KEYWORDS</u>
alienation ~ Connection
scattered ~ Centered
hoarding ~ Sharing

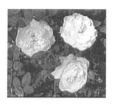

This day, do only one thing.
Surrender to Love.
It is the deepest longing of your soul.

Loving Relationships
Rosa 'Tineke'
Harebell Flower

This formula helps to deepen self-love as well as the love and acceptance of others, encouraging one to release the *strings attached* conditions one places on relationships.

Have you ever been in a relationship in which you expect absolutely nothing in return—one that was completely unconditional? No strings attached? Chances are good the answer is no.

We are socialized to create relationships with all kinds of strings attached. A baby cries and then gets food. As we grow, we trade our friendship for emotional and social acceptance; job performance for money and a sense of security; seek romantic relationships in order to feel worthy and loved. All the while we've been dangling from a bunch of strings, either manipulating or being manipulated by others.

This essence formula helps us to become aware of these binding strings, begin to detach from them and to create healthier relationships.

The crystal-white bloom of *'Tineke'* rose brings the message, "I am worthy of love just as I am", encouraging one to experience and share love in all of its purity and beauty.

Harebell flower catalyzes one's ability to give and receive love unconditionally.

Pattern of Imbalance: Feelings of low self-worth that are projected onto others; victim role; placing unrealistic demands on self and others; perfectionism, over-achieving, never good enough.

Affirmation
**I allow myself to receive and to give love unconditionally.
I release all attachments.**

KEYWORDS
over-demanding ~ Genuinely Accepting and Appreciative
perfectionist ~ Flexible
attached to outcomes ~ Healthy Detachment

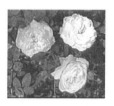

*Open your heart to God's Love -
no matter what.*

Open Heart
Rosa 'Fair Bianca'
Mesquite Flower

*T*his formula fosters sincerity, serenity and peace. It inspires the opening of the heart.

This transformation of the heart is ultimately facilitated by God's Spirit and can be supported by this beautiful white rose, *'Fair Bianca'*. Gold-white is a color that symbolizes a connection with God and unity with Christ.

Mesquite flower warms the heart, amplifying the quality of the body's life-force energy needed during such an opening.

Pattern of Imbalance: Insincere, self-absorbed, unwilling or unable to show compassion towards others.

Affirmation
**I am serene. I am at peace.
Within my heart awakens tenderness, compassion and the highest expression of love.**

KEYWORDS
insincere ~ Sincere
self-absorbed ~ Empathetic
self-serving ~ Compassionate

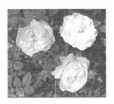

Within your essence, within your soul lie the seeds of all possibility.
Take care of those seeds. Nurture them.
Love yourself.

Self-Love & Peace
Rosa 'Tiffany'
French Marigold and Iris Flowers

*T*his essence formula gently comforts and nourishes the heart, aiding in the process of releasing suppressed feelings and memories of past hurts. It fosters self-forgiveness and acceptance. Through this nurturing process, a deeper inner peace is realized and self-fulfillment is promised. May also be used before and during stressful situations to bring inner calm.

The light pink color of *'Tiffany'* rose brings sweetness, gratitude, appreciation, admiration and sympathy, all qualities that are found when one is able to forgive oneself, and others, and be fulfilled.

Yellow, the color of the base of *'Tiffany'* rose, offers enjoyment in the moment and friendship with oneself. It is also associated with the solar plexus and the quality of acceptance of one's life and one's sense of self-expression.

Iris flower helps us to find peace and meaning in life, while French Marigold helps us to hear that still, small voice of promise within that encourages a sense of inner peace.

Pattern of Imbalance: Self-hatred, loathing, anger turned inward causing inner turmoil, lack of self-nurturing, self-abandonment.

63

Affirmation
**I now accept and love myself unconditionally.
I am at peace within.**

KEYWORDS

turmoil ~ Calm
self-abandonment ~ Self-Nurture
agitated ~ Meditative
anxiety ~ Calm in the Present Moment

Gary's Story: From Anxiety to Inner Peace

Gary was dreading a trip to the east coast. This caused him to experience a lot of anxiety. He was flying back to appear in court for a hearing that could potentially affect his job and career. His wife had tried some essences and had found them helpful, so he called me and asked for a formula to help him with the stress he was feeling.

I prepared *Self-Love & Peace* formula for him at stock level and advised him to take four drops twice a day. The following day he left on his trip. When Gary returned a week later, he was amazed at how peaceful he had felt throughout his ordeal. He'd started the essence formula as soon as he received it and took several drops three times daily during his trip. While on the plane, he said affirmations and was able to feel less anxiety and get focused as he prepared his court deposition. He took the essence before he appeared at the hearing at which he calmly gave his deposition. The court ruled in his favor. He returned from his trip feeling tranquil, at peace and relieved that the ordeal had not been as stressful as he'd feared it would be. He felt greatly supported by this essence formula.

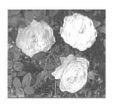

So, put to sleep the fears, the anguish and the pain.
Cultivate the earth of your heart.
Fertilize it.
Plant caring seeds and experience God's immeasurable
love.

Self-Nurture
Rosa 'Sea Pearl'
Mariposa Lily and Lavender Flowers

Like the discovery of the pearl within the newly opened shell, this formula helps one discover the still, quiet, nurturing inner voice of God's Spirit and recover one's own preciousness and beauty.

Sometimes, we become so preoccupied with activity in order to avoid negative feelings that we burn the candle at both ends. This, of course, means we'll experience the inevitable burnout.

The rose, 'Sea Pearl', with its lovely apricot-pink vibration, brings nurturing to the heart. This rose also supports the hardiness and resilience we need to eventually bounce back from having carried trauma around for so long. It allows us to reconnect through the heart to that quiet, nurturing voice within.

Mariposa Lily flower helps us to deal with the grief of having lost touch with the joy and innocence of our child-self and to reconnect with her, while Lavender flower aids in calming and balancing emotions when we are over-extended.

Pattern of Imbalance: Negative feelings toward self; always on the run; burned out.

Affirmation
I acknowledge and attend to all of my needs.
I lovingly nurture myself.

<u>KEYWORDS</u>
burnout ~ Nurturance
self-negativity ~ Self-Appreciation

Melinda's Story: Easing Out of Perfectionism and Burnout

Melinda had been an overachiever and perfectionist since she was a teenager. She'd gotten to a point in her life when she was just tired of trying to do everything and do it perfectly all the time. Working two jobs and running a business were just not working for her.

Exhausted and depressed, she obtained this formula with hope that it would help to ease her oppressive feelings. She took the essence once a day for 6 weeks and allowed herself to take a vacation. She found that she could relax and enjoy spending time with her family and friends, read magazines and watch old movies that she dearly loved without feeling guilty that she should be doing something more productive in her eyes. When she returned from her vacation, she resolved not to continue at one of her jobs so that she'd have more time to do the things she loved, which included writing and painting.

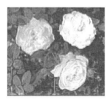

*Let love radiate from within you,
as you cherish and share the
magnificent life you have been given.*

Share Love
Rosa 'Cherish'
Shooting Star Flower

*T*his essence formula helps one to appreciate one's inner gifts and to expand outwardly with them.

Contemplating the name of the rose, '*Cherish*,' in this combination formula is a key to understanding the workings of this essence. When we cherish something, it holds deep meaning for us. The deeper the meaning attached to something, the more apt we are to be willing to love it unconditionally and to express this love.

The soft, coral-pink color of this rose, '*Cherish*', and Shooting Star flower support the movement of love's light outward from the place of sharing our God-given gifts, assisting us to radiate love without thinking about it, spontaneously and without judgment.

Pattern of Imbalance: Placing conditions on one's experience of love, self-focused

Affirmation
**I allow myself to receive and to give love unconditionally.
I release all attachments.**

<u>KEYWORDS</u>
conditional love ~ Unconditional love
judgmental ~ Accepting

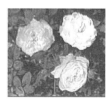

Stress Rescue – Five-Roses Formula
Rosas: 'Altissimo', 'Fair Bianca', 'Pristine', 'Regatta', 'Summer Fashion', Self-Heal and Dandelion Flowers

*T*his combination formula assists with extreme feelings of overwhelm, stress and burnout. The balancing and nurturing qualities of the five roses, when combined, balance all of the energy centers, help to "smooth out" the emotions and promote resilience and endurance.

The vital energy is balanced as loving energies of the roses in this formula calm and open the heart to the nurturing inner voice and help to shift our conscious awareness, fostering a greater sense of calm, centeredness, grounding and equilibrium in our body.

Self-Heal and Dandelion flowers help to anchor the healing energies of the roses into the emotional and physical bodies.

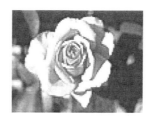

CHAPTER 7
HOW TO CHOOSE YOUR
PERSONAL HEALING ESSENCES

W hen choosing rose flower essences for personal healing, you may prefer to use one or more of the following methods. With practice you will discover which method(s) work best for you.

Asking for Higher Guidance

While you are self-healing with rose flower remedies, you are working at the spiritual and soul levels. So, it is quite appropriate, and even desirable, to ask God's Spirit to guide you as to what you truly need. God knows your true essence and what would benefit you the most. Here are a few suggestions for preparing to ask for Higher Guidance:

1. Find a quiet time and place and meditate or pray about your challenges and which essences might assist in your healing.

2. Hold each essence bottle in your hands or lap and sense its subtle energies.

3. Now ask silently, or aloud, "Is this essence right for me at this time?" Remain open to receive an answer. You may choose to utter a prayer or simply ask the question. The answer my come as a feeling, a sensation, a voice or image.

4. Flow with it. Trust in God's guidance. Group each essence that you are guided to use together, separating them from the rest. You may later wish to write down your impressions in a journal. How you do this is ultimately up to you.

5. Give thanks to God for guiding you.

Acknowledging Your Positive Potentials and Spiritual Aspirations

You may choose your healing essences by recognizing and acknowledging your aspirations (positive spiritual qualities you wish to seed and nurture within yourself), such as self-love, compassion, patience, sincerity, etc. Here's what to do:

1. Go outside to your garden, a quiet space in nature or find a quiet indoor space away from distractions. If outdoors, listen to the sounds of nature. If indoors, play relaxing music. Visualize yourself in a beautiful location out in nature that is calming and relaxing. Experience the vivid colors, sounds and sensations all around you.

2. Get into a quiet, meditative state by breathing deeply and calming your body and mind.

3. Shift your awareness and begin to imagine yourself in certain situations or circumstances in your life and how you would behave, react, respond, in them. For example: You may see yourself in an argument with a family member who is very hurt and crying, knowing that you would normally react in a very hurtful, resentful and defensive way towards them.

4. Begin to visualize and *feel* yourself listening to their side of the story, acknowledging their feelings, hugging each other, calmly walking away arm-in-arm, etc.

5.   Acknowledge how you *aspire* to *be* in this situation: *patient, compassionate, giving, forgiving.* Stay with these images and feelings as long as you can.

6.   Write down these aspirations, images and feelings in your journal as they come to you or record them on a cassette or CD so you can replay them as reminders later.

Go through steps 4, 5 and 6 as many times as you wish in order to get a good self-assessment and to help you choose the rose flower essence(s) that will best support you. Visualize yourself as loving, successful, happy, healthy, etc., and *feel* the qualities within you that allow and support you to *be what you aspire to be.* These qualities correspond to specific rose flower essences. Write them down.

7.   Choose the rose flower essence(s) or formula(s) whose descriptions include or closely match your list of aspirations.

8.   Acquire or hand-make the essences you have chosen. See Chapter Nine, "How to Make Your Own Rose Flower Essences".

9.   After you have begun taking the essences, make time to continue to do the visualization exercises as well as to speak, write, or even sing affirmations to help anchor into your subconscious these images, feelings and positive qualities you aspire to express from your deepest heart. When in the actual situations, choose to react differently, supported by your work with the rose flower essences.

10. Give thanks for the process.

Now that you've acknowledged your positive potentials, you may wish to choose one of the following methods to hone in on which essences will most help you.

Scanning Your Body for Unresolved Feelings

Most of us tend to be out of touch with our true feelings most of the time. In essence, we numb ourselves into a state of *not feeling*, and act/react from a false persona or personality. Women, in particular, have been culturally trained to do this— to hide the *bad* feelings of anger or hurt or sadness in order to take care of their children, partners, or friends. Men do the same in order to appear *strong* and *in control*.

The body has an amazing ability to store memories and feelings. Many feelings have not been expressed through the emotions. The habitual suppression of emotions causes imbalances in the body's energy system that can eventually manifest as emotional and mental unrest, pain and disease.

You can learn to scan you body to identify areas of tension and pain in order to become aware of underlying feelings. Once you connect with these feelings, you will be able to choose a flower essence or formula to address them. Scanning your body to help you choose your rose flower essences may take some practice, but will prove to be quite rewarding. When you connect with how you *truly feel,* you begin the process of uncovering the *true you* that is hidden beneath blocked and unresolved feelings. How long the process takes depends upon just how deeply you've buried your true self. Rose flower essences can help you to work through, resolve and release painful feelings, and free you to be more fully actualized in your life rather than resigned to it.

To begin to scan your body for your feelings:

1. Sit quietly and comfortably. Begin to progressively deepen your breathing, as it is comfortable for you.

2. Focus attention on your body. Notice any areas where you feel stress, tension, discomfort or pain. Concentrate on each area and *ask that area (organs, muscles and tissues) to tell you what the pain or discomfort is about. Listen to your body. It will speak to you. And it doesn't lie.*

3. Without censoring, jot down or digitally record the answers as you ask questions aloud to each part of your body. You may be very surprised at what you find. Be gentle and accepting of yourself as these answers are revealed to you.

Most likely, your body will zoom right in on what is *really* going on. It will probably be specific enough that you will easily find essences or formulas in the repertory in this book that correspond to the imbalances or issues for that area.

4. If you find that your answers aren't clear when you've finished this asking process, look up the corresponding body energy centers and organs in Appendix D (e.g. stomach pain corresponds with solar plexus area, which corresponds with unexpressed emotions, poor boundaries, etc.) and choose an essence or formula that corresponds to those imbalances.

5. Thank your body for assisting and guiding you.

Using Muscle Checking (Kinesiology)

Kinesiology, or muscle testing as it is commonly called, is another way to choose essences. A client recently brought to my attention that the word "test" has negative connotations for her, causing her muscles to tense and her breathing to shut down. So, I prefer to call this muscle-testing technique, *muscle checking*.

It is best to muscle-check yourself with the assistance of an experienced flower essence practitioner, who has a variety of rose flower essences on hand, to help you to choose your essences. Here is the procedure:

1. Hold out your writing arm, stiffly to the side, perfectly parallel to the floor. Resist as your partner (the flower essence practitioner) pushes down on your arm close to the wrist. This is the *default* check. Unless you are ill or fatigued, or your partner is a sumo wrestler, you should respond with enough strength to maintain a strong resistance.

2. Next, (and this is where it gets interesting), put into your non-dominant hand a food that you may be allergic to or a substance, such as tobacco or white sugar, that generally weakens the body. Hold it against your solar plexus (stomach/spleen area). Resist again as your partner pushes down on your other arm. The majority of people experience a slight electrical "short circuit" in the body's energy system and the arm muscles weaken. You should notice that your arm is initially less able to resist as your partner pushes down. This is the *negative* check.

3. Muscle check for each rose flower essence bottle you have on hand, having your partner push the arm down as you hold each bottle next to your solar plexus. If the essence is appropriate, you shouldn't notice any changes in the arm muscle's strength. If the essence is inappropriate, you will notice a marked weakness.

Sometimes the weakness is very slight, so you will have to be observant and have a scale of some sort: a *yes* category for essences for which the muscle stays strong; a *no* category for essences to reject because the muscle responds by weakening; and a *maybe* or *neutral* category for essences which don't seem to clearly be either *yes* or *no*.

Once you've gone through several essences, a few should indicate "yes". You may choose from these essences for your healing program. There is usually no need to try thirty essences before deciding on one that's right for you.

With an occasional client I have found that all of the essences check as *no* or *neutral*. This usually indicates that this form of assessment may be inappropriate and that the person may respond more readily to another method of choosing essences or to another healing modality. It may also mean that essences just aren't appropriate for that person *on that day*. It's best to try again tomorrow.

Using the Keywords and Repertory

The most intellectual, non-physical and non-intuitive method of choosing rose flower essences without the aid of a professional flower essence practitioner is by checking the keywords and the repertory, each rose flower essence description found in Chapter Eight, and by finding the pattern of imbalance that the formula addresses or the positive healing qualities the essence supports.

An optimal approach for choosing rose flower essences for self-care would be to combine two or three of the methods mentioned and cross check the results. Most likely, you will find that many of the same essences show up in the final checklist.

Various Ways to Take Rose Flower Essences

There are several ways to take your rose flower essences. The most common way is by mouth, but topical application, bath immersion and application via mist-spray are also very effective.

After using any combination of the spiritual, intuitive or intellectual methods discussed (prayer or meditation for guidance; acknowledging your aspirations; scanning your body for your feelings; muscle checking; using the repertories and keywords), you may take a few drops of the chosen essences or formulas. It would be best to start with only one or two essences at a time. However, if you wish to take more essences, you may muscle check to find appropriate groupings of essences or formulas to take simultaneously. You may also decide to combine several essences in another dosage bottle. Follow the directions for "How to Prepare a Dosage Essence" in Chapter Nine.

When taking an essence, place 4–7 drops under the tongue or put a few drops into a glass of water, juice or herbal tea and sip over a period of time during the day. Never allow the dropper to touch your mouth or tongue. This will assure that the dropper remains sanitary and free from bacteria that would contaminate your remedy.

can apply the rose flower essences to the body energy ᴧters that are listed in the essence descriptions or the chart in Appendix A. You can also mist spray the essences around your body or enjoy them as additives in a relaxing bath.

CHAPTER 8
THE REPERTORIES

*T*he repertory is a quick way of finding a rose flower essence according to the imbalance(s) it addresses.

You can also find an essence by tuning in to positive soul qualities you aspire to nurture within yourself (aspirations). Then, find that quality as listed in the repertory to see which essence or formula is associated with it.

You may check back under the rose flower essence and formula profiles before settling on an essence or formula, just to make sure that it is the one you wish to take.

Rose Flower Essence Repertory

To discourage focusing on the negative, this repertory purposely does not have a listing of qualities according to negative behaviors or imbalances. Instead, it focuses upon their opposites. For example, if, after scanning your feelings, you become aware of inner turmoil, then you may decide to choose an essence that supports *calm* or *peace* or if you are experiencing conflict with another person, you may choose an essence that supports *cooperation*. Tune in to your soul's highest positive aspirations in order to choose and work with the rose flower essences.

When there is more than one rose flower listed, you may choose one essence or use them in combination.

According to Positive Aspiration
pire to be, to embody, to express

Adaptability – 'Anastasia', 'Sea Pearl'
Adoration (sincere) – 'Royal Wedding'
Align and Energize Subtle Energy System – 'Eglantine', 'Tournament of Roses'
Aromatherapist – 'Royal Dane'
Artist Within (manifest) – 'Jayne Austin'
Balance – 'Pristine', 'Regatta', 'Tournament of Roses'
Beauty (love of) – 'Bride', 'Fair Bianca', 'Summer Fashion'
Calm – 'Bill Warriner', 'Pristine'
Celestial Music (attunement to) – 'Paul Shirville'
Centered – 'Camara', 'Elizabeth Taylor', 'Pristine'
Charity (sense of) – 'Perdita'
Cherishing of Things Dear – 'Cherish'
Child-Like Spirit – 'Anastasia'
Clarity (mental) – 'Melody Parfumee'
Clarity of Understanding in Love – 'Harlequin'
Co-Existence Among Species (peaceful) – 'Evelyn'
Compassion – 'Guy de Maupassant'
Composer – 'Paul Shirville'
Confidence – 'Camara', 'Summer's Kiss'
Contemplation – 'Elizabeth Taylor'
Contentment – 'French Perfume', 'Summer's Kiss'
Cooperation Among Species – 'Evelyn'
Courage – 'Lanvin'
Creativity (harmonize with) – 'Anastasia', 'Jayne Austin', 'Regatta'
Culinary Enjoyment – 'Royal Dane'
Curiosity (heartfelt) – 'Tamora'
Dance (supports) – 'Anastasia', 'Louise Odier'
Delight (in simple things) – 'Double Delight'
Devotion – 'Royal Wedding'
Discovery (sense of) – 'Tamora'
Divine Potential – 'Brandy'
Emotional Change (positive) – 'Arizona', 'Y'ves Piaget'
Empathy – 'Guy de Maupassant'

Endurance (supports physical) – 'Crystalline', 'Grand Impression'

Energy (increased) – 'Perdita'

Enthusiasm – 'Pat Austin'

Equilibrium – 'Bill Warriner'

Exercise (prepare for) – 'Grand Expression'

Faith – 'Perdita'

Feeling (sense of deep) – 'Summer's Kiss'

Five Senses (energized, stimulated) – 'Chrysler Imperial', 'Summer Fashion'

Focus – 'Granada'

Forgiveness – 'Guy de Maupassant'

Fulfillment (deep) – 'Brass Band'

Gladness – 'Y'ves Piaget'

Goals (spiritual) – 'Brandy'

Gratitude – 'Bride', 'Madame Isaac Pereire'

Grounding – 'Mister Lincoln'

Growth (spiritual, enthusiasm for) – 'Pat Austin'

Happiness (Innate) – 'French Perfume'

Hardiness – 'Sea Pearl'

Harmony – 'Crystalline'

Healer (supports) – 'Sunset Celebration'

Healing (emotional) – 'Fragrant Plum', 'Y'ves Piaget'

Healing (physical) – 'Altissimo', 'Eglantine', 'Pat Austin'

Healing Environments (create in nature) – 'Pat Austin'

Higher Purpose – 'Gertrude Jekyll'

Hope – 'Perdita'

Infinite Source (connection with) – 'Madame Isaac Periere'

Innocence (child-like) – 'Anastasia', 'Just Joey'

Inventor – 'Tamora'

Joy – 'Just Joey', 'Summer's Kiss', 'Touch of Class', 'Y'ves Piaget'

Laughter – 'Summer's Kiss', 'Touch of Class'

Life Transitions (understanding) – 'Granada'

Love (aspiration for true) – 'Double Delight', 'Madame Isaac Periere', 'Mon Cheri'

Love (awareness of) – 'Madame. Isaac Pereire'

Love (sharing of) – 'Cherish', 'Evelyn', 'Teneke'

Love (unconditional love) – 'Cherish', 'Evelyn'

Love (understanding underlying pattern) – 'Harlequin'

Meditation (moving) – 'Elizabeth Taylor'
Meridians (energized) – 'Chrysler Imperial'
Moment (enjoyment of) – 'Tiffany'
Motivation – 'LD Braithwaite'
Musician – 'Paul Shirville'
Nature (love of) – 'Bride', 'Timeless'
Nervous System (help to balance) – 'Pristine'
Optimism (heartfelt) – 'Louise Odier'
Patience – 'Y'ves Piaget'
Peaceful – 'Bonica', 'Camara'
Perception (heightened) – 'Pristine'
Perseverance (encourage) – 'Sea Pearl'
Purity of Love (sharing of) 'Tineke',
Quietness – 'Fragrant Plum'
Release Inner Energy – 'Yves Piaget'
Relationships (deepen) – 'Timeless'
Resiliance – 'Sea Pearl'
Responsible Inter-Species Co-Habitation – 'Guy de Maupassant'
Reverie – 'Bill Warriner'
Rhythms (attunement to) – 'Bill Warriner', 'Electron', 'Paul Shirville'
Sanctuary – 'Bill Warriner'
Self-Appreciation – 'Sea Pearl'
Self-Confidence – 'Sea Pearl'
Self-Expression – 'Regatta'
Self-Friendship – 'Tiffany'
Self-Generation – 'LD Braithwaite'
Self-Healing (encourage) – 'Altissimo'
Self-Honor – 'Gertrude Jekyll'
Self-Love – 'Tiffany', 'Timeless'
Self-Value – 'Tineke'
Serenity – 'Pristine'
Service (sense of destiny for) – 'Evelyn', 'Tiffany', 'Timeless'
Sincerity – 'Timeless'
Singer, Singing Voice – 'Fair Bianca'
Smell (enhance sense of) – 'Royal Dane'
Spiritual Dimensions (perceiving) – 'Mon Cheri', 'Pristine'
Spiritual Growth – 'Pat Austin'

Spiritual Insight (deepen) – 'Pristine'
Spiritual Reality (deepen) – 'Crystalline'
Spontaneity – 'Touch of Class'
Stillness – 'Fragrant Plum'
Stress (endure, cope with) – 'Altissimo', 'Just Joey', Stress Rescue 5-Rose Formula
Subtle energies (awareness of) – 'Fragrant Plum'
Surrender (spiritual) – 'Royal Wedding'
Talents (lovingly share with others) – 'Sunset Celebration'
Tenderness – 'Tiffany'
Tranquility – 'Bill Warriner'
Trust – 'Summer's Kiss'
Unity (inner) – 'Double Delight'
Wellbeing (greater sense of) – 'Eglantine'
Wonder (sense of) – 'Just Joey'

According to Rose Name

'Altissimo' – healing (physical), stress (endure, cope with)
'Anastasia' – adaptability, creativity, child-like innocence, dance (supports)
'Arizona' – positive emotional change
'Bill Warriner' – calm, equilibrium, reverie, tranquility, sanctuary, attune to subtle rhythms
'Bonica' – peace
'Brandy' – goals (spiritual), divine potential
'Brass Band' – fulfillment
'Bride' – beauty, simplicity (appreciation and love of)
'Camara' – centering, gaining confidence, peace, joy
'Cherish' – cherish things dear, share love unconditionally
'Chrysler Imperial' – energize five senses and meridians
'Crystalline' – harmony, deepen spiritual reality
'Double Delight' – delight in simple things, true love (aspiration for), unity (desire for)
'Eglantine' – bio-energy system (align), well-being (greater sense of), healing (physical)
'Electron' – rhythms (attune to subtle)
'Elizabeth Taylor' – centering, contemplation, moving meditation
'Evelyn' – peaceful co-existence/cooperation (desire for), service (sense of destiny for)
'Fair Bianca' – beauty (love of), singer, singing voice
'Fragrant Plum' – awareness of subtle energies, encourages stillness, healing
'French Perfume' – contentment, happiness
'Gertrude Jekyll' – self-honor, higher purpose (seek)
'Granada' – life transitions (understanding)
'Grand Impression' – endurance (supports physical)
'Guy de Maupassant' – compassion, empathy, forgiveness
'Harlequin' – clarity of understanding with love
'Jayne Austin' – artist within (nurture)
'Just Joey' – wonder (sense of), innocence (child-like), joy
'LD Braithwaite' – motivation, self-generation
'Lanvin' – courage
'Louise Odier' – dance, (supports), optimism (heartfelt)

'Madame Isaac Pereire' – awareness of love, gratitude
'Melody Parfumee' – clarity (mental)
'Mister Lincoln' – grounding (when spacey)
'Mon Cheri' – aspiration for/ awareness of true love, spiritual dimensions (perceiving)
'Pat Austin' – enthusiasm, healing environments (create), healing (physical), spiritual growth
'Paul Shirville' – celestial music (attune to), composer, musician, rhythms (attune to)
'Perdita' – charity, faith, hope, (sense of)
'Pristine' – serenity, deepen spiritual insight, heightened perception, balance nervous system
'Regatta' – balance, creativity, self-expression
'Royal Dane' – aromatherapist, culinary enjoyment, smell (enhance sense of)
'Royal Wedding' – adoration (sincere), spiritual devotion
'Sea Pearl' – adaptability, hardiness, perseverance, resilience, self-appreciation, self-confidence
'Summer Fashion' – five senses (energize, stimulate)
'Summer's Kiss' – contentment, feeling (deep), joy, laughter, trust
'Sunset Celebration' – caregiver, healer, talents, (lovingly share with others)
'Tamora' – curiosity (heartfelt), discovery (sense of), inventor
'Tiffany' – enjoy the moment, self-friendship, self-love, service (sense of destiny for)
'Timeless' – love of nature, self-love, service, sincerity
'Tineke' – purity of love (sharing), self-value
'Touch of Class' – joy, spontaneity
'Tournament of Roses' – alignment and balancing of subtle energy systems
'Y'ves Piaget' – emotional healing, patience, release energy, joy and gladness

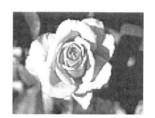

CHAPTER 9
HOW TO MAKE YOUR OWN
ROSE FLOWER ESSENCES

*I*n order to prepare a healing rose flower essence, you must be truly inspired. Working with these wonderful healing allies is a deeply spiritual exercise. You must be attuned to their subtle energies and committed to work with them with the utmost integrity, love and respect.

If you are feeling called to make your own rose flower essences for self-healing or to offer to your family and friends then, by all means, do it!

The Sun Method

Have you have ever watched the morning dew form on the flowers in your garden with the morning sunrise? If you have, you've witnessed nature's method of making flower essences. An alchemical interaction occurs among these forces—earth (the flowering plant), air, fire (the sun's light and energy) and water—that creates the healing flower essence.

Animals, birds and insects love to drink the dew from flowering plants. They instinctively know that it is healing for them.

You can closely imitate nature's method of making rose flower essences by using the sun method. All you need is an open heart, a bit of patience and a few inexpensive utensils. Here's how to begin:

1. Sit or recline near the plant in its natural habitat or in your own organic garden and quietly attune yourself to its beauty and to your natural surroundings.

2. Make sure that you are clear and sincere in your intentions about healing with the essences. Offer a prayer to communicate your intentions. In this way, you are asking permission to be a co-creator of healing with God's healing agents, the plants.

3. You will need a sterilized clear glass or quartz crystal bowl. Avoid using lead crystal. It will negatively affect the flower essence. Quartz is preferred, as it is nearly a pristine clear, vibrational container for the essence. It will naturally help to purify and amplify the subtle energies of the essence contained within. You can sterilize your bowls by washing them in very gentle dish soap, then rinsing them well in warm water. Fill the clean bowl three-quarters full with pure spring water.

4. Choose a rose blossom or several blossoms that are near their highest maturity. Remember, the plant is sacrificing a beautiful part of itself, so be sure to be sensitive as you harvest. You may feel guided to cut a few blossoms or just one. Be careful not to touch the blossom or stem with your bare hands and introduce bacteria. Wear clean, soft, white cotton or linen gloves or use a clean white piece of cotton or linen to handle the severed stem and blossom or handle them with a leaf plucked from the stem.

5. Visually check the upper side of the blossom closely for small insects, (green aphids or black thrips), that may be residing in the petals. Also inspect the underside for insect egg sacs or webbing. You may be able to brush them away if there are only a few, but if the amounts are fairly large, choose another blossom.

6. Clip the rose blossom at the stem using a small, clean pair of scissors or a pincher. I prefer to use quartz crystal rods to

pinch and sever the blossoms from the stems. The quartz helps to prevent shock to the plant and does not introduce the energy of any metal to this delicate process.

7.   Float the rose blossom(s) on the water in the bowl.

8.   Optional: Cover the bowl with a clear glass or quartz crystal lid or a clean swatch of white cotton or linen if you wish to keep out bugs and other organic substances, which may fall into the essence and contaminate it. Secure it by wrapping a rubber band around the cloth and the rim of the bowl if it is windy. The sun's rays will still penetrate the cloth as well as the glass.

9.   Place the bowl in the full light of the morning sun as close to the mother plant as possible in order to vibrationally transfer as much of the plant's life-force energy to the essence as possible. Leave the bowl in the morning sun for several hours until noon. This is when the sun's rays carry the most life-force energy that will alchemically imprint the healing signature of the flower blossoms into the molecular matrix of the water, creating the flower essence.

10. Prepare the mother essence as described below in the section "How to Prepare the Mother Essence."

The Moon Method

Moonlight is a soft reflection of the sun's light. Naturally, it may also be used to create your rose flower essences. The moon's light imparts an effect to flower essences that seems to work more deeply in the realm of the subconscious aspect of the human psyche. In the case of rose essences, white roses seem to best respond to the cool, milky white light of the moon. I encourage you to experiment with making essences in moonlight with other roses and flowers and to test their results.

The method is identical to that of the sun method with one exception. Since the light of the moon waxes and wanes, it is best to expose the blossoms in the bowl of water to the light of the *full* moon for several hours during the night, until just before dawn. It is also possible to make an essence while the moonlight is in its waxing or waning phase, but the light will not be as intense and the essence may not be as potent. When the process is complete, prepare the mother essence as described in the section "How to Prepare the Mother Essence."

The Boiling Method

In the 1930s Dr. Bach boiled many of his flower specimens (including Wild Rose) to make his mother essences. To prepare an essence using this method:

1. Place your flower blossoms in a clean enamel pot (preferred) or stainless steel pot partially filled with pure spring water. Never use an aluminum pot. A glass, pyrex pot may also be appropriate.

2. Bring the water and blossoms to a gentle boil. If stems and leaves are included with the blossoms, boil without the lid for 30 minutes. If only the blossoms or petals are present, gently boil without the lid for 15 minutes. Let cool.

3. Pour the resulting liquid off into another enamel or glass container, straining through cheesecloth or an unbleached coffee filter to eliminate any organic materials.

4. Prepare the mother essence as described in the section "How to Prepare the Mother Essence" later in this chapter.

Alternative Methods of Preparing the Essence to Prevent Plant Trauma

If, like me, you are very sensitive to inflicting suffering, you'll want to prepare your flower essences using less invasive methods. With these methods, a plant can be spared the trauma of being cut and its life force can be fully preserved while making rose flower essences. Some of these methods require a little ingenuity and patience. They are:

A. Place the blossom, still attached to the plant, within a clean glass or quartz bulb that contains the spring water. The bulb's opening will have to be large enough for the blossom to pass through without damage. Expose to the full morning sun.

B. Situate the still-attached blossom in half of a crystal geode that contains spring water and expose to the full morning sun.

C. Situate the still-attached blossom in a bowl of spring water and expose to the morning sun. In order to do this, you may have to use string or other props to position the blossom correctly in the water. Be careful not to damage or break the petals or the stem.

D. Sit next to the plant. Go into a deep prayer and ask God's Spirit and Nature for permission and guidance to co-create a healing essence with the plant. Then ask in prayer that the plant's healing energies be transferred to the water. Once you are certain that permission has been granted, wait until the plant transfers its healing energies to the water sitting in the bowl nearby. This process can take from several minutes to an hour.

Proceed to preserve and bottle the mother essence as described below.

How to Prepare the Mother Essence

Once your rose flower essence has finished steeping, you will make what is known as the *mother essence or mother tincture*. This is the bottled essence that you will preserve, store and from which you will make your stock strength and dosage strength essences.

1. You will probably see little bubbles that have formed on the inner walls of the glass or crystal bowl when you return to

your bowl at noon (sun method) or dawn (moon method). This is formed, in part, due to the alchemical process that has taken place. The healing energies of the flower have been imprinted within the molecular makeup of the water via the action of light of the sun and the forces of nature. In essence, the water now carries the *vibrational memory* of the flower blossom.

2. Remove the blossom from the bowl by scooping it up with a sterilized glass cup. Deposit it back upon the ground near the mother plant.

3. Pour the transformed water through a clean piece of cheesecloth, cotton cloth or unbleached coffee filter into a sterilized amber, cobalt or violet bottle half-full of 80-proof vodka or brandy (available from your local liquor store). This 50/50 ratio of water to alcohol preserves the essence and deters bacterial growth. You can use one, two or four-oz. dropper bottles that you have purchased and sterilized for this purpose. Sources are listed in the Resources section. You can also use recycled amber vitamin bottles that you have washed and boil-sterilized. Tightly cap the bottle. Label with the name of the rose followed by the words "mother essence" and the date. You now have your rose flower mother essence.

If you are sensitive to alcohol, as an alternative stabilizer and preservative you can use apple cider vinegar or *red shiso (Red Shiso Perilla Frutescens)*, an herb commonly used in Japanese cuisine. Sources for *red shiso* are listed in the Resources section.

4. Place the mother essence on the earth near the mother plant (out of sunlight) for a couple of hours to anchor and potentize the flower essence. You can also potentize the essence by vigorously tapping it against the palm of your hand several times. Store in a cool, dark place until you are ready to prepare your stock strength and dosage strength essences.

If the essence is for personal use, you can forego the use of a preservative altogether. When I started making flower essences for myself, this was my approach. It does, however, increase the chance that the essence will spoil, especially if it contains any organic material. If you opt not to use a preservative, store the tightly closed essence bottle in the refrigerator in a brown or black paper bag to deter bacterial growth and to avoid degradation by the artificial light bulb. Be advised that without the stabilizing and preserving agent, the flower essence may begin to lose its purity and potency, so you should use up the essence within a couple of weeks. Discard the essence if you notice any bacterial growth.

To prepare a flower essence for ingestion, you can dilute the mother essence to the stock level and then to the dosage level based on your needs.

How to Prepare a Stock Essence

1. Fill a sterilized, ½ or 1-ounce amber, cobalt blue or violet glass dropper bottle half-full with brandy or vodka. Apple cider vinegar or *red shiso* may also be used.

2. Using a clean glass dropper, take 7 drops of the mother essence and place them into the bottle. Top off with spring water. One may also use clustered water, a special processed water that may be substituted for spring water in any of the essence-making processes described in this book. (See Glossary and Healing Therapies Contact Information for more information on clustered water).

3. Cap the bottle with the glass dropper top and attach an identification label.

4. Store in a cool, dark place.

5. When ready, ingest 1–2 drops at a time, three times a day, or more often when needed.

6. Return to storage space when not in use.

How to Prepare a Dosage Essence

1.   Fill a sterilized, 1/2-oz. or 1-ounce amber, cobalt blue or violet glass dropper bottle one-quarter full with brandy, vodka, *red shiso,* or food-grade vegetable glycerin (available at health-food stores.)

2.   Place 7 drops of the *stock essence* into the bottle. Top off with spring or clustered water.

3.   Cap the bottle with the glass dropper top and label it.

4.   Offer a prayer of gratitude for this genuine healing gift.

5.   When ready to use, ingest 4–7 drops at a time, three times a day, or more often when needed.

6.   Store in a cool, dark place when not in use.

How to Prepare a Rose Flower Essence Formula

You can prepare and use a rose flower essence formula much in the same way that you would a single essence. The only difference is that, instead of adding 7 drops of a single stock essence, you add 2–4 drops of the stock essence of each flower to the quarter-full dropper bottle of brandy, vodka, or *red shiso,* It is advisable to limit a rose flower essence formula to perhaps two to three types of roses or other flowers. Top off with spring water, as you would a single flower essence.

How to Prepare a Rose Flower Essence Mist Spray

To prepare a rose flower essence mist spray:

1.   Take a sterilized 1-oz. amber, cobalt blue or violet bottle with a mist spray pump top and fill it one–quarter full with brandy or vodka. See the Resources section for sources of these types of bottle.

2.   Add 7 drops from the stock bottle of your favorite rose flower essence.

3.   Top off with spring water and seal with mist spray pump top.

4.   Optional: Add a couple drops of your favorite pure essential oil for added fragrance and healing benefits. Remember to shake the bottle vigorously to disperse the oil throughout the carrier solution before spraying. Be careful to avoid spraying near the eyes.

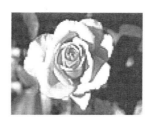

CHAPTER 10
BATH THERAPIES WITH ROSE FLOWER ESSENCES

*B*athing in water infused with rose flower essences is an excellent way to infuse your cells and your bio-energy system with their healing energies. You can add essential oils, whose healing qualities complement those of the rose flower essences, to your bath for a heightened healing and fragrant experience.

Rose Flower Essence Bath Therapy
and Aroma-Massage

Bath time is a wonderful time to work with rose flower essences. What other time during the day do you consider complete down time - away from people, the phone and your daily worries? During a soothing rose flower essence bath you can let go of the stresses of the day. As you gradually relax and become more introspective, you set the stage for the rose flower essences to do their healing work.

To prepare your therapeutic bath:

1. Add each rose flower essence formula to your bath water: 4 drops for stock strength, 7 drops or a full dropper of dosage strength. Add to warm bath water as it is running and stir in spirals.

97

2. Add 3–5 drops each of the essential oils that have been blended together in a teaspoon of jojoba or massage oil.

3. Continue to swirl the water until blended.

4. You may also add a drop or two of the oils to an aromatherapy diffuser to infuse and saturate the air with their fragrances while you bathe.

During your relaxing aromatic essence bath, absorb the energies of the rose flower essences through your body's pores for 15 minutes. Gently massage your body, working from your feet upwards to release tension and soothe pain. Afterwards, bathe with rose, jasmine, rosewood or lavender soap.

You can substitute less-expensive rosewater for rose essential oil in recipes where it is called for. See the Resources section for sources of pure essential oils, rosewater and other hydrosols.

Do not use the essential oils if you are pregnant, lactating or asthmatic without first consulting your health care professional.

Essential Oils and their Latin Names:
Cedarwood – *Cedrus atlantica, Juniperas virginiana, Cedrus libani*
Chamomile – *Matricaria recutita, Anthemis nobilis*
Clary Sage – *Salvia sclarea*
Fennel (Sweet) – *Foeniculum vulgare dulce*
Frankincense – *Boswellia carterii*
Jasmine – *Jasminum officinale, J. grandiflorum, J. sambac*
Lavender – *Lavendula amgustifolia, L. officinalis*
Mandarin – *Citrus reticulata, C. nobilis*
Marjoram (Sweet) – *Origanum majorana*
Myrrh – *Commiphora myrrha*
Rose Otto – *Rosa damascena*
Rosemary – *Rosmarinus officinalis*
Rosewood – *Aniba rosaeodora*
Sandalwood – *Santalum album*
Ylang Ylang – *Cananga odorata*

Rose Flower Essence Aromatherapy Baths

Compassion ~ Forgiveness Bath

Compassion ~ Forgiveness and *Self-Love & Peace* formulas, rose and rosemary essential oils, or clary sage/fennel blend for bath, diffuser or aroma-massage.

Expression of Love

Love's Expression formula, rose, lavender, clary sage essential oils for bath, diffuser or aroma-massage.

Faith in the Storm Bath

Faith in the Storm formula, rose, frankincense (by diffuser), mandarin essential oils also for diffuser or aroma-massage.

Grief Relief Bath

Self-Nurture and Grief Relief formulas, rose, lavender, marjoram essential oils for bath, diffuser or aroma-massage.

Heart Balance Bath

Heart Balance formula, rose, lavender, jasmine and rosewood essential oils for bath, diffuser or aroma-massage.

Lightness of Heart Bath

Lightness of Heart formula, rose, lavender, jasmine essential oils for bath, diffuser or aroma-massage

Love Source Bath

Love Source formula, rose, lavender, rosemary essential oils for bath, myrrh and sandalwood oils (by diffuser) for divine inspiration. You can substitute ylang ylang, or sandalwood-cedarwood blend to the diffuser for contemplation and meditation. Myrrh-sandalwood blend is best for prayer.

Loving Relationships Bath

Loving Relationships and *Compassion ~ Forgiveness* formulas, rose, lavender, clary sage essential oil for bath, diffuser or aroma-massage.

Open Heart Bath

Heart Balance and *Open Heart* formulas, rose, lavender, jasmine essential oil for bath, diffuser or aroma-massage.

Self-Love & Peace Bath

Self-Love & Peace and *Self-Nurture* formulas, rose, lavender, chamomile essential oils for bath, diffuser or aroma-massage.

Self-Nurture Bath

Self-Nurture and *Self-Love & Peace* formulas, rose and lavender essential oils for bath, diffuser, or aroma-massage.

Share Love Bath

Love's Expression and *Share Love* formulas, rose, lavender, jasmine essential oils for bath, diffuser or aroma-massage.

The *Grief Relief*
Stone Massage Aromatherapy Bath

Gather the following before beginning your stone massage aromatherapy bath:

Candle (Natural-Aromatherapy preferred)

Essential Oil(s) 5 drops rose and 4 drops lavender essential oils for bath

Grief Relief formula

Seven - ½ inch sculpted massage stones (See Resources section for sources):

Bloodstone
Rose Quartz
Rose Quartz point
Amethyst
Clear Quartz point
Seraphinite
Obsidian point

Now to begin:

1. Light your favorite aromatherapy candle or put a drop or two of each essential oil into your aromatherapy diffuser.

2. Run a warm bath. Add a dropper-full *Grief Release* formula as well and one full of the rose/lavender essential oil blend. Stir into bath water with a figure-8 motion.

3. Put on your favorite relaxing music.

4. Step into the tub and soak.

5. Begin to breathe deeply, from down low in your abdomen.

6. With thumbs and knuckles, rub the web of skin between your thumb and first finger of each hand. If this area is tender, you are probably holding onto grief in your heart center and lung area. Continue to rub gently as you breathe and notice any sensations, thoughts or feelings you may have.

7. With both thumbs, rub the back of each thigh and calf, careful to notice the tender spots and lines (meridians.) Follow the meridians intuitively.

8. Continue to breathe deeply. Select the bloodstone and massage. Use an upward motion to rub the back of your thighs and calves of your left leg with a rounded end of the stone. The oils in the bath water will help the stone glide more readily over your skin. You may find yourself following the meridians that are tender, (probably the gall bladder, kidney, spleen and liver meridians).

9. Starting at the center, begin rubbing the sole of your left foot with the smooth, rounded end of the stone, using vertical strokes and small circular motions. You may feel bumpy or grainy areas, particularly in the arch of the foot. These areas correspond to your solar plexus - your stomach, spleen, liver and diaphragm - which may be holding onto blocked energy, particularly if you haven't been able to express anger or cry recently. Massage here with deep breathing, allowing the *Grief Relief* rose essence formula to be absorbed through the pores of your skin and into your energy meridians. This will greatly help you to begin to release this unwanted negative energy.

10. Continue to breathe deeply—inhaling through the nose, exhaling through the mouth—as you apply massage to areas of the sole of the foot with small, circular movements.

11. Switch to the rounded rose quartz massage stone and repeat on your right foot.

12. Switch to the rose quartz pointed stone and begin to gently press into the sole of your foot. I like to think of this as a form of *pointed stone acupressure*. At this point, if you have continued breathing deeply, you will probably feel small releases—your digestion may open up, you may feel releases in your neck and jaw and you may even begin to cry.

Your diaphragm may begin to move up and down and tears may well up in your eyes. Allow yourself this release, without judging or intellectualizing, as you continue your breathing. Remember, your body is letting go of age-old blockages that have been obstacles to your optimum health, wellbeing and full self-expression. You may find yourself passing gas, belching or making other sounds. Your abdominal muscles and solar plexus are releasing the tension and pressure held there.

13. Continue, repeating the above with each of the other stones on the list in the order that they appear. If you feel that you want to omit or substitute other stones or to follow another order, that's fine. Feel free to follow your intuition.

14. After the release is complete, center yourself and calm your breathing. Sit quietly to assimilate the meaning of the release then give thanks for the healing process.

15. Complete and enjoy your bath.

16. After your bath, you may wish to record the experience, your feelings and thoughts in your journal.

17. Give thanks for your healing.

A Personal Experience with Flower Essence Bath Therapy

Notes from a springtime bath:

This morning I woke up feeling pretty awful. My jaw is tight and painful and I am worrying about bills, the writing of my book, my business and my day job. My thoughts seem to be spinning out of control, but I know it is emotional. I am feeling overwhelmed.

What to do? I think I could jump into my car and drive out to some remote desert area about 20 miles away and scream my head off. Instead, I decide to take my Sunday morning bath therapy session.

I postpone my usual fruit and herbal tea breakfast for later and start to run the bath. I stir a dropper-full of *Self-Love & Peace* formula into the water along with an essential oil blend of lavender and rose in cocoa butter bath oil. As its lovely scent wafts among the tiles, I light a votive candle and place a bar of rosewood soap with rose petals on the side of the tub next to the five massage stones that I use for foot reflexology therapy.

I slide into the tub to soothing music. The music's underwater theme, with its dolphin and whale songs, is mesmerizing.

My jaw, neck and shoulders throb. My diaphragm feels tight. I know I need a release. The three smoothed and arched massage stones (bloodstone, rose quartz, amethyst) on the edge of the tub sit next to the rose quartz and clear quartz points. I begin to massage the soles of my feet with each stone, one by one, first the left foot, then the right. As I press the point of the rose quartz stone into the heel of my left foot, my diaphragm releases and the tears began to softly flow. I realize that I am tired of working so hard and want my mommy. These are the feelings that are finally coming to the surface.

Switching to the right foot, I know that a deeper release is on its way. When I massage the arch of this foot, it always triggers a deep release and cleansing. This time I'm not disappointed. I find myself weeping, as the rose-quartz massage technique combined with that of the rose flower essence formula and the essential oils, opens a part of me to let go and heal the pain. As I cry, I feel the tension in my jaw intensify for a few moments until the end of the release. I know that this is the discomfort I awakened with this morning. Finally, the tension is released and my jaw relaxes.

Feeling much better, I say a prayer of thanks for the release, blow out the candle, bathe and wash my hair. I emerge, free of the unresolved pain and overwhelming feelings, replaced with a sense of hope and optimism. I feel lighter and cleansed and more prepared to take on the challenges of the day.

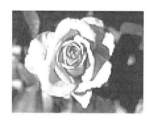

CHAPTER 11
OBSERVATIONS BY ESSENCE USERS

*M*any users of the rose flower essences have shared their healing experiences via my Rose Essence Research Program (formerly under the auspices of Crystal Radiance). These essences seem to inspire subtle, yet important shifts in feelings and thoughts.

Ørjan Repaal, iridologist, homeopath and homotoxicologist whose practice is in the ABC klinikken in Oslo, Norway:

Repaal, who works extensively with vibrational remedies and is very sensitive to them, tested five separate rose essences on himself with the following observations:

'Double Delight' – "Gave me the feeling of warm love. I felt happy, and I got a sensation of joy. I feel an effect to the heart."

'Evelyn' – "I felt a clearness of mind, and a concentrated feeling, determination and an effect to the pituitary gland with an improvement of intuition."

'French Perfume' – "I felt sadness and slightly depressed. Things appeared to be difficult. After some minutes I got a sensation of burnout, and some interference with the spine pulse to the brain. It gave me an effect to the nervous system, merely the CNS."

'French Perfume' (repeat use) – "I've used 'French Perfume' for myself occasionally when I get a "burnout" feeling, and I can feel my brain pulse improve in seconds!"

Author's comment: It seems that Repaal's first experience with the **'French Perfume'** rose flower essence brought up the negative state of burnout. However, once that negative state was identified, the same essence addressed the issue and catalyzed a noticeable positive improvement with subsequent use. This is a common occurrence with flower essences.

'Guy de Maupassant' – "Like the **'Double Delight'**, this essence gave me a feeling of warm love. While the former gave a distinct joy, this essence gave me a more satisfaction – a feeling of being happy and satisfied, an effect to the heart."

'Tiffany' – "It felt like my thoughts ended, thinking and concentration got very slow. I started to brood and ponder. It gave me an effect to the brain somehow, probably the frontal cerebellum area."

When Repaal used rose flower essences with his clients, he reported:

Girl, 16 years old:
Difficult childhood. Mother drug addicted. Now living with her father and his wife. Complained of loss of menses, digestive problems, loss of appetite, diarrhea. Used **'Guy de Maupassant'** for four weeks - Digestive problems disappeared. Appetite improved. Still has loss of menses. Feeling happier.

Woman, 48 years old:
Deep depression. Slight anxiety. Tiredness. Digestive problems, heartburn. Divorced from her husband. Headaches, muscle aches. Neck and shoulder tension. Sclerosis. Using Zoloft (anti-depressive-Pharmacia), and Zantac (digestive Pharmacia).

Used **'Double Delight'** and **'Tiffany'** rose flower essences, 20 drops, 2 times a day for 4 weeks. She also took homeo-toxologic remedies. After taking the remedies for four weeks, she has had muscle pain and headaches (related to Mucokehl, a homeopathic remedy from Sanum). She has not noticed any changes on the mental/emotional level. (Things do go slowly, of course, when the patient is using Neuro Pharmacia [antidepressant]. But her appearance is more *radiant* and her eyes hold more *life* somehow).

Woman, 42 years old:
Cold childhood. Needy. Needs approval. Afraid of rejection. Tends to hyperactivity. Easily stressed. Took **'Tiffany'** and **'Double Delight'** for four weeks - The summer with her mother has gone surprisingly smoothly. Not perfect, but she hadn't the need to confront her.

Nine weeks later, she took **'Tiffany'** and **'Guy de Maupassant':** She then had a strong reaction to the remedy. She called me and felt down, depressed and touchy. I told her to continue the essence and told her that this was an outburst of negative emotions and that relief would come later on.

Woman, 37 years old:
Bad childhood. Alcoholic father. Traditionally had bad self-feeling (low self-esteem) and identity problems. Difficult understanding of what is normal and abnormal between alcoholics and children.

She's got a lot of treatment, but in September during taking **'Tiffany'** rose essence, she called me just to tell me how wonderful she felt, and that she has planned to write a book with a fictitious person based on her life.

Woman, 32 years old:
Several lighter complaints.
After taking **'Evelyn'** rose flower essence she claimed that her relationship with her daughter had improved.

Observations by Other Users of the Rose Flower Essences

'**Pat Austin**' – "I've been using '**Pat Austin**' once a week, and I noticed an immediate and deep shift... I can say that **Pat Austin** [rose essence] has been helpful...I test to take the rose essence only about one time a week." *Massachusetts*

'**Fragrant Plum**' essence – "This week I began with a trip to my doctor (D.O., Acupuncturist, Herbalist). I was experiencing a very painful back, which he and I believe is sciatica. The treatment was wonderful! Never before has my back pain been relieved while the acupuncture needles are inserted. I felt really great. But Thursday morning, I felt the pain again. I also examined my mind and found that I felt overwhelmed. As usual, there was too much to do and way too little time. So, I took the essence that morning. I went from having pain any time I bent over slightly in the garden, very early in the morning, to feeling great by the time I went to work." *Arizona*

'**Anastasia**' – "Second day using the essence I felt very feminine and pretty. The third day hit hard! Very sad, almost overwhelming (not depression) – sad, painful memories came up - particularly when I was a young girl - stuff I had forgotten about. This continued through the third week. The fourth week, felt more calm, relaxed, less stressed." *Utah*

'**Mon Cheri**' – "Heart opening, specifically to romantic love possibilities, also, sensitivity to memories and releasing grief around romantic love experiences. Appreciation of what *is* sensuality without really wanting more. I can definitely feel the effects of the rose essence. There is a deep love-opening happening inside me, perhaps as deep as the red of '**Mon Cheri**'. The romantic in me is certainly awakened, but there is much more than this. It is with a love for greater humanity, and with more compassion and sensitivity that my heart awakens." *North Carolina*

'**Sea Pearl**' rose essence, which is contained in *Self-Nurture* flower essence formula – "So far one of my favorite essences has been

110

Self Nurture. What an impact this essence played in my everyday life! I could not believe that on my days off I really tested (kinesiology) for a lot more drops…I guess the reason for this was because I am a massage therapist and I am booked for a year… So on the weekends I found that this essence helped me to take time for me to self-nurture me and I did just that. I really think I found I had far more energy using this essence on the weekend to do what I needed to do, but also had time to pamper myself!" *Ohio*

'Tiffany' rose essence, which is contained in *Self-Love & Peace* formula – "I have really made some progressive-positive changes (using *Self-Love & Peace* formula) in my life. I really believe that the tincture has helped me to focus and to stay in the moment. I have especially utilized the tincture to help me surface my suppressed emotions that hold back my growth. I firmly believe that using tools such as flower essences is very helpful…" *Arizona*

'Y'ves Piaget' – "I was afraid of opening to love. I am noticing a heart opening that is slow and subtle, yet a perceptible and wonderful process. I feel softening and awakening in my heart center, my sensitivities are perhaps a little heightened emotionally, yet in a safe and flowing way." *North Carolina*

'Evelyn' – "My observations of this (**'Evelyn'**) essence were that it affected my root and sacral energy centers – issues of family were pushed to the surface to be released. I felt grounded in my own power, not caught up in old family dynamics. It seemed to keep my heart open in the process also. Felt very nice, warm, pinkish light from the essence." *Minnesota*

'LD Braithwaite' – "I tested to start this essence tonight. Immediate impressions with first dose: Flattened out extremes of emotion. Brought about a more middle range: highs and lows, but smaller amplitude. I've been having some symptoms of upper respiratory allergy or low-grade infection w/slight sore throat and earache the past few days. This essence energy seems to have gone right to my ears – my ear (esp. left) seems very clear…

Right hand— very hot at first. Then arm. Then arm and right shoulder, working up into the ear. Quieter mind…" *Massachusetts*

A woman who tested via kinesiology to take 'Y'ves Piaget' essence four times a day for a month – "I found that the areas of my spine seemed to really be affected in the sacrum area. All areas stayed in place much better." *Ohio*

'Tineke' rose essence, which is contained in *Loving Relationships* formula – "I feel like the *[Loving Relationships Formula]* essence is having an effect… like something is taking hold. I feel like the fragments are floating closer together and when they come within range of each other, they'll come together like the piece of a puzzle. I feel so strong inside myself today…like something deep and powerful is happening on my insides…" *Arizona*

A man using a custom formula combining: 'Fair Bianca', 'French Perfume', 'Pat Austin', determined by muscle checking – "I definitely felt more joyful and enthusiastic. I'd like more! I stopped using it for a few weeks and I did notice that when I got back on it, that the enthusiasm was a nice surprise and the most dominant." *Arizona*

'Anastasia' rose essence, which is contained in *Lightness of Heart* formula – 'I feel so much more focused and clear." *Arizona*

'Tiffany' rose essence, which is contained in *Self-Love & Peace* formula, – 4 drops orally, three times daily for four months - "I was very disheartened by my girlfriend of eight years when our relationship was in question. Needless to say, I was brokenhearted and I allowed this essence to help me keep my heart open. These essences are the most healing that I have encountered. We managed to stay connected and I attribute it to my determination and the essence." *Texas*

A woman on a very clear and committed healing program, taking the following formulas over a four month period – *Self-Love & Peace* formula, which contains 'Tiffany' rose essence; *Grief Relief* formula, which contains 'Double Delight' rose essence; *Loving*

Relationships formula, which contains **'Tineke'** rose essence states:

"I have found the essences help me to focus, take a few moments to meditate, affirm myself several times a day. I have incorporated the affirmations into my daily meditative, healing practices. They have helped me to move through and process issues I've been dealing with and they have greatly helped me affirm and accept my love for myself and my appreciation for all I receive in my life." *Arizona*

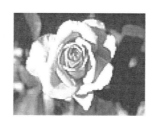

CHAPTER 12
OBSERVATIONS BY A
LaStone™ Massage Therapist

*U*sing rose flower essences in conjunction with massage therapy can bring additional benefits to the experience. Yvonne, a massage therapist from Great Britain who practices LaStone™ Massage Therapy, shares this account of her use of *Self-Nurture* formula, which contains **'Sea Pearl'** rose essence. This essence can help one with self- appreciation, self-nurture and resilience.

Yvonne says:

"I tried using it, (*Self-Nurture* formula) in the water with the stones and didn't really feel there was anything happening on a level that I could see or feel. Nor did I have any real response from my clients. I then put several drops in my oil. This is when I started to notice a difference.

"One elderly woman, who I see on a regular basis for a back massage (no stones), seemed to respond better to the massage, or should I say that her muscles and body seemed to release their knots and tension easier and with less work on my part. I did do some silent sound work with her as well. At the end of the massages she seems to be happier within herself and has less complaints when I go to see her. She has even started to schedule a massage more frequently!

"Another client, [in her] early thirties, who came for stress and tension and then stopped coming for a period started back again. I was using the essences when she came back—we used both stones and just hands— she appears calmer within herself, more grounded, more in touch…and all of this even though she is going through some stressful times at work and home.

"Whereas before, my clients enjoyed their massages, now, in a way in which I can't always put my finger on, they seem to enjoy the massage even more and seem contented on a different level. When I have used oils without the essences, for some reason there is a difference in their reaction. It may also be, and I am sure this is the case, a response within myself as I have the oil and essence on my hands."

CHAPTER 13
A LaStone ™ Therapist's Journal

S ue, another LaStone™ Massage therapist, who lives in Wisconsin, shares a journal of her use of **'Anastasia'** rose flower essence over a seven and a half – week period. This beautifully displays how a rose flower essence can work over time to gently support, heal and balance in one's daily life. The journal has been lightly edited for space, continuity and relevance.

Journal

10-19   During massage I felt more energy flowing and I felt guided to the clients' needs as I used stones in my regular massage sessions.

10-20   Nothing too noticeable this day.

10-21   Took **'Anastasia'** essence under my tongue the night before and woke up very sensitive under my tongue and throat. It lasted most of the day.

10-22   Studied for the National Exam. All of my thoughts involved studying and knowing I will pass, I was able to think very positive.

10-23   I was very calm for taking the National Exam. I was thrilled that I passed and did very well in all categories. I have a good feeling of completion. My thoughts were positive to move on to complete other tasks in my life.

10-24   I enjoyed a beautiful orange moon with my husband and twin boys. I felt closeness in the moment but yet a little sad and I'm not sure why.

10-25   I felt [so] overwhelmed at the things that needed to be taken care of that I put [them] off because of work and studying.

10-26   I felt a little sad about the ten-year anniversary of my brother's death. I took the opportunity to be able to celebrate happy memories of his life throughout the day, which helped me elevate my mood.

10-27   I am feeling calm in my mind not to worry about what doesn't get done. There is always another day.

10-28   I felt good to have time to myself in the evening. I was able to put my mind at rest. I began using the **'Anastasia'** essence in a spray bottle with essential oils before each client's massage. They noticed the uplifting scent, but I noticed too that they could feel the energy but couldn't describe it.

10-29   I was very tired this day. I had to drive two and a half hours in a car to our cabin with my mother-in-law. She is a very negative and energy-draining person. The essence, I believe, helped me to be in a calm, almost numb state…

10-30   I had an energetic day with lighthearted ambition to complete a project. I didn't let negative thoughts enter my mind.

10-31   Very mentally draining day as my mother-in-law played negative mind games. I let it affect me and forgot to take the **'Anastasia'** essence [until] after the fact. I felt calmer in the evening after I remembered to take the essence. I was able to dismiss the hurtful comments [and prevent them] from entering my energy field.

11-1   I was overwhelmed at all the tasks that I wanted to complete. As I continued to take the **'Anastasia'** essence, I was able to break the tasks into smaller pieces and felt good about all that I accomplished. I did not let the things that I did not complete haunt my mind.

11-2   I am still using **'Anastasia'** essence in a spray bottle in my treatment room. I am feeling clients relax more and leave with a peaceful mind and body.

11-3   Since I began using **'Anastasia'** essence during my massage, I have had more clients coming to see me. Many repeat clients. Coincidence? I had an emotional breakdown in the evening with my family. I felt everyone was taking me for granted and didn't realize all that I do for them or the sacrifices I make for them. Finally, when I think I will be able to receive someone's kindness, I become disappointed because it was never intended for me. My husband often doesn't think of my needs and wants. Instead, he is too busy taking from me. I had to cry and release to realize that I bring this on myself. Only I am responsible to take care of myself. I should not expect others to think of doing anything for me. Therefore, I will take care of myself and only do for others when I want to. I need to learn to say no when that is what I want to say.

11-4   I feel better emotionally. Even regular massage feels so much more guided when I spray the essence in the room.

11-5   I had a headache early in the day. I kept taking **'Anastasia'** essence continuously as I felt I needed to. I was happy and playful in the evening.

11-6   I was very energetic. I am now putting **'Anastasia'** essence in my water daily besides under my tongue in the morning and evening.

11-7 I am still very energetic and feel very at peace. I was at our cabin in the woods. I conducted a funeral for past hurtful events. Mary Nelson [the founder of LaStone Therapy™] suggested this for a traumatic period of my life that I had trouble letting go of. I lit a candle, burnt a paper of the hurtful event and the people and place involved listed on the paper with a few choice words as to how I felt toward a certain person. I buried the ashes along with some stones in the ground by a big pine tree. I feel much better. It is in the past and buried.

11-8 This day almost felt like an accomplishment day. I spent most of my time finishing up unfinished business and I felt very good about that.

11-12 I am thinking about leaving my job ... I am beginning to feel taken advantage of and not being compensated properly for my healing work. I will draw strength from the essences to face my employer and tell her how I feel.

11-13 I can still feel so much energy in my treatments with the stones as I use the essence in a spray. The clients can feel it too and comment, but are not sure what it is.

11-14 A lot of thoughts are clouding my head in regards to finding happiness in my career.

- I confronted my employer about the misunderstanding in my employment agreement as to how I should be paid. I pretty much am getting $10.00 an hour. She became very defensive and I was extremely emotional. I couldn't stop crying for several hours. I just kept taking **'Anastasia'** until I felt peaceful. I received a LaStone™ [massage] treatment. I took the essence throughout the day to see what I would feel. I know I reached a meditative state very quickly and felt at home with the stones placed on me.

- Things seem to be happening fast. I felt very confident in myself as I interviewed for a job in Green Bay. They offered me a position immediately with 50% commission during massage and $7.00 an hour when not in treatments. I talked to my employer about leaving. She tried to top my new offer but I felt it was too late. I need to be closer to my home and family. My job was in another city and the commute was becoming too much for the small wages I was making. Also, my sitter quit and I now have no one to watch my boys after school. Being in Green Bay would allow me to be more flexible.

- Clients continue to comment on how different my massage is. They say something along the lines of "One of the best massages they ever had" or "There is something different about you… you are really good" or "How long have you been doing this? You are really good. There is just something about you!" I am just flattered at the wonderful comments and I feel it is the energy work they are feeling. The essences definitely enhance the energy. The evening was one of female bonding. I was energized to be with my friends and had a lot of fun.

11-15 through 11-28   I must combine this very confusing week. I was seeking guidance on my decision where to go with my career. Both of my children were sick on different days. One of the days was my birthday so I couldn't do anything but take care of him. The other day one was sick during a family get-together for my birthday and I had to miss that too. I drew strength from the essences…

- I have decided to open my own practice in a new salon…I have listed many options and decided to give this one a try. I am also interviewing at a place to work one day a week. I need the exposure and some other source of income along with my line and flower essences.

-   I feel like I am in a spinning top and I am waiting for it to stop. I am very busy making up brochures and new business cards so when I leave my position [at my current job], I will have clients at my new business. I am mostly taking **'Anastasia'** essence...

-   I am feeling on top of the world. This is the last day at [my present job] for the most part. I will still return to work with clients that have bought packages with me.

12-5   I am taking relaxation time for these two days to give me strength to begin my new business venture.

12-6   Devastation! The people I was supposed to rent from didn't sign my contract as they said they were going to after I changed one thing on it, otherwise we were set to go. They said I could move all of my things in and begin today (as I did just that). One of the owners got a call from someone recently that offered them more money for the space. Now I either have to match that offer or lose the money I already invested in brochures, business cards, newspaper ads, etc. They felt they could do this because they had not all signed the contract. I decided they were not the type of people I wanted to do business with. So I will be out of $400.00 plus. I would rather cut my losses and move on. The day got better when I got home and my husband's chiropractor was on my answering machine offering me space in his practice.

12-13   I...decided to begin orally taking **'Anastasia'** again. I went back to my oil painting and needed the flow of my artistic ability.

Summary

I have noticed a vibrational difference in not only myself, but in my treatments with clients as well. I will be making use of the essences in all of my treatments either by room spray, topical, or introducing them to clients for oral use. (I would like to further study them before recommending them for oral use to clients.) I feel **'Anastasia'** brought on a realization that I needed to move forward with my career as a massage therapist.

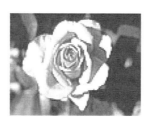

CHAPTER 14
BIOFEEDBACK IMAGING REVEALS
BIO-ENERGY CHANGES

*T*he rose flower essences are intimately involved with the bio-energy field and energy centers of the body in the process of healing.

Computer software interpretations of biofeedback imaging photography show effects of rose flower essences on the energy centers and bio-energy field when ingested or placed at the base of the neck and spine. The biofeedback device produces an electronic interpretation of the bio-energy field by measuring the electrical potential along meridian points of the palm of the hands of each volunteer. It then converts the information to an electrical frequency and displays this as colors and patterns over the figure. The meaning of the colors is based upon different electrical measurements. Each color has a measurable electrical frequency.

Biofeedback imaging photography offers compelling evidence that some type of activity is indeed taking place within the body's energy centers and the bio-energy field when these remedies are taken. The author and five volunteers took rose flower essences orally or applied the essences topically. Neither the author nor the volunteers knew which essence they were taking at the time, although all consented to participate. The following accounts detail how the biofeedback device interpreted the changes they experienced.

1. The Author- unknown essence administered to her by Donna Crystal, bio-feedback imaging specialist

When I ingested a full dropper of the hybrid tea rose essence, **'Fair Bianca'** (not known to me at the time), the biofeedback imaging device showed changes in my bio-energy field and energy centers after ninety seconds.

In the video and computer print-outs my bio-energy field showed a dramatic shift, from appearing primarily turquoise-blue in color, with the sacrum, solar plexus and heart energy centers appearing yellow-green, to showing a deep magenta coloring, centered around the heart and throat areas. The color affected the first four energy centers - deepening and amplifying the red in the root energy center particularly, while shifting the next three energy centers to more orange in color. There was a dramatic shift in the throat energy center - it appeared more prominent and a deeper blue. The halo of the bio-energy field changed, shifting from green, closer to the shoulder area, to violet, with green at the outer portion of the field over the right shoulder and to the left of the left hand and foot.

Interpretation: The sacral, solar plexus and heart energy centers changed from yellow-green to deep magenta, centering over the heart center. The bio-energy field and energy centers shifted from a social, communicative helping mode (turquoise-blue) to an intermediate intellectual-yellow learning, creative mode to finally, a more grounded, energetic state with the vital force expressing itself in the root and heart areas. The throat energy center deepened in blue, its natural color, suggesting that the energy here increased, perhaps becoming more balanced. The shift in the bio-energy field from green to violet suggests a shift to being in a more calm, balanced, spiritual/healing state.

'Fair Bianca' is an essence that brings nurturing to the heart and encourages a deeper self-expression. The biofeedback imaging results seem to confirm these healing qualities.

126

2. Marilyn

When Marilyn orally ingested the rose flower essence **'Fair Bianca'**, and also had it topically applied to the base of her spine (root energy center), the video and her computer print-out showed that her bio-energy field shifted from a soft turquoise-blue with green over the right shoulder and around the left hand and foot, to a more bluish field with indigo blending in at the perimeters over the left shoulder and around the right arm and hand. The energy halo around the head shifted from a greenish-blue to a whitish-blue, and it expanded upwards. The heart energy center seemed to expand, and to become more intensely yellow-green.

Interpretation: Marilyn's bio-energy field changed from soft turquoise blue with green (social, communicative) to blue-indigo suggests a shift to a more introspective, calm intuitive state. The heart center expanded and intensified in color, suggesting more energy at this center. The change in the halo from green-blue to blue-white with upward expansion suggests a shift to an extended state of heightened spiritual awareness.

'Fair Bianca' is an essence that encourages a deeper spiritual nurturance to the heart. The biofeedback imaging results seem to confirm these healing qualities.

When Marilyn orally ingested a full dropper of *Stress Rescue* formula, which at the time contained the four roses, **'Fair Bianca', 'Altissimo', 'Regatta',** and **'Summer Fashion'** and had it topically applied to the base of her spine, the video and computerized printout indicated changes. This implies that there were dramatic changes in her energy centers and bio-energy field.

Interpretation: The most immediate and dramatic shift appeared in Marilyn's bio energy field. It showed a considerable expansion, which could indicate an increase in her vital energy. Secondly, it shifted away from indigo and turquoise blue to yellow-green, with the brightest part at the base of the right foot and around the calves, as well as around the head, which shifted dramatically in color from light blue to yellow-green. This halo of color around

127

the head also expanded, along with the general expansion of the bio-energy field.

Stress Rescue formula seemed to initially cause an energizing effect upon the energy field. Perhaps this, for Marilyn, was a preliminary step towards reducing stress.

3. Liliana

When Liliana was first connected to the biofeedback-imaging device, her bio-energy field appeared on the printout and in the video as predominantly orange-yellow, with more yellow on the left side. There was a bit of yellow concentrated on the right side. There was a concentration of orange above her head also.

After she took a full dropper of the rose essence **'Madame Isaac Pereire',** there was a noticeable shift in the color of her bio-energy field above her head to the green-blue range. The concentration of orange became turquoise-blue and was much larger.

Interpretation: The orange and yellow colors present in the bio-energy field when Liliana was first connected to the biofeedback device indicate a bright intellect, active life-force and a creative personality. Liliana is energetic and has a lot of inner strength. When the colors shifted after she ingested the rose flower essence to a light and deep green and blue – it indicated an inflowing of harmony, peace and warmth.

'Madame Isaac Pereire' rose flower essence seemed to support and deepen positive attributes of Liliana's soul as well as foster a sense of peace and wellbeing.

4. Cephias, (Liliana's son, 4 years old)

Cephias really wanted to try the rose flower essence and the biofeedback-imaging device, so his mom let him! *Heart Balance* formula, containing **'Fair Bianca'** rose essence was administered: 2 drops on the backs of both hands, 1 drop at the nape of the neck, 1 drop at the base of the spine (root center). Cephias also insisted on holding the bottle for a moment in both hands.

Initially, Cephias' energy field was filled with green in the center with yellow and orange appearing around the inner green circle. His energy centers were visible on the printout – the first three being the brightest. After taking *Heart Balance* formula, which contains **'Fair Bianca'** rose essence, there was a dramatic shift, particularly in the energy centers. They appeared much larger and the upper centers brightened considerably. A purple glow surrounded Cephias' heart center. The entire bio-energy field turned to indigo-blue. There was also a turquoise glow above his head.

Interpretation: Cephias is a beautiful child who is very comfortable playing and exploring outside in nature. He has many creative ideas, which he joyfully shares with all of his friends of any age. He is very bright, loving and articulate. These are qualities that the colors green and yellow indicate on the biofeedback image printout prior to taking the rose flower essence. After taking the rose flower essence formula, there seems to have been an affect on all of the energy centers, with the heart center being affected in a particular way – it emanated a purple glow. The turquoise blue and indigo colors in the bio-energy field indicated an inflow of harmony and peace as well as a stronger spiritual state.

Heart Balance formula seemed to support Cephias to grow in trust and harmony.

5. Alesha

Alesha's biofeedback photo and video initially showed her bio-energy field as turquoise blue with a magenta pink section to the right from her brow to her foot and on the left side from her heart to the soles of her feet. Her energy centers showed a soft glow, with a purple glow at the crown and a green tint around the heart and throat. After taking the **'Evelyn'** flower essence, Alesha's bio-energy field became almost uniformly turquoise-blue with a white tint throughout. Her energy centers intensified in brightness and color.

Interpretation: Alesha is an artist and writer, very dedicated to her quest for learning and sharing knowledge with others. **'Evelyn'** rose flower essence seemed to energize her bio-energy centers, particularly the root, sacral, throat and brow. Perhaps the essence strengthened her artistic and aesthetic sensibilities and communicative abilities as a teacher as it supported her solar plexus, heart and throat centers.

'Evelyn' rose flower essence seems to support these positive qualities of Alesha's soul so that she may use her talents and abilities to live for the service of others.

6. Richard

When Richard arrived, his bio-energy field showed on the biofeedback printout as red and orange with yellow on the left side. His body's energy centers were visible in the photo, except the throat and crown. After taking **Fragrant Plum'** rose flower essence and waiting several minutes, the bio-energy field and energy centers appeared the same as before. There was no discernable change during this session.

Richard was the only volunteer whose biofeedback information showed little or no change after taking a rose flower essence during the session.

These biofeedback images and data imply that there is activity and influence exerted upon the bio-energy field as well as upon the energy centers when rose flower essences or formulas are ingested orally and/or applied topically to the base of the neck and spine, major test points for flower essences. Additional research may offer concrete evidence of these effects in the future. See Appendix E for a transcript of Tenanche's and Marilyn's sessions.

ENDNOTES

Endnotes to Chapter One

1. Vasudeva Barnao, "The Wildflowers of Australia – Living Essences of Australia" *Essences of Nature Magazine, Vol. 3, Issue 3, p. 26.*
2. Clare G. Harvey, Amanda Cochrane, *The Encyclopaedia of Flower Remedies,* p. 5.
3. Vasudeva. p. 26.

Endnotes to Chapter Two

1. G. Brennan, *Easy Roses* (Chronicle Books, 1995), p. 14.
2. The rose's ability to assist us in "keeping it all together" during major life spiritual and emotional transitions is easily understood when we see how Vitamin C, found in rose hips, works at the cellular level. It acts as "glue", keeping our cells and tissues cohesive. Vitamin C keeps us from literally falling apart. U. Erasmus states in *Fats that Heal, Fats that Kill* (Alive Books, 1993), pp. 70-71:

> "Vitamin C plays several key roles in the human body. It *is required for the synthesis of the 'glue' that* surrounds our cells (mucopoly-saccharides), makes them cohesive, and keeps our tissues from falling apart and landing on the floor in a pile of individual cells. In this role, vitamin C is important for tissue integrity and the prevention of invasion by foreign organisms and cancer cells."

"Vitamin C is *necessary for the production of the proteins collagen and elastin* (specifically, the hydroxylation of the amino acids lysine and proline), which keep our arteries, bones, teeth, cartilage, scar tissue, and other tissues strong. Lack of vitamin C (scurvy) results in weakened arteries and bleeding into tissue spaces."

3. J. Lawless, *Rose Oil* (Thorson's, 1995), p. 12.
4. J. Lawless, *Rose Oil* (Thorson's, 1995), p. 14.
5. Dr. Leonard Perry, *"Rose Hips"*.
www.backyardgardener.com/masterg/rosehips.html
6. J. Balch, Phyllis A. Balch, *Prescription for Nutritional Healing* (Avery Penguin Putnam, 2000), p.43; *"Lycopene: The Rediscovered Carotene"*, *Life Extension Magazine*, *Aug. 1999, p. 1,* ((http://www.lef.org/magazine/mag99/aug99-report1.html):

"Lycopene is an open-chain unsaturated carotenoid that gives the red color to tomatoes, guava, watermelon and pink grapefruit [and rose hips.] In the body, lycopene is deposited in the liver, lungs, prostate gland, colon and skin. Its concentration in body tissues tends to be higher than all other carotenoids. Lycopene scavenges free radicals more efficiently than Beta-Carotene. Current research suggests that lycopene's antioxidant properties provide a high degree of protection against heart disease caused by high cholesterol and may also boost immune function by increasing natural killer cell activity in the body." (The Olympian Labs, Inc. Product Reference Guide.)

7. Dr. Philip M. Chancellor, *Bach Flower Remedies*, pp. 223-24; Nora Weeks, *The Medical Discoveries of Edward Bach, Physician*, p. 128.
8. J. Lawless, *Rose Oil, p. 35;* P. Davis; *An A-Z Aromatherapy, pp. 277-78; Bruce Berkowsky, "The Soul Nature of Rose Oil", Massage and Bodywork, June/July 2002, pp. 58-59.* Additionally, in my meditations and musings about the rose's healing signature, I have theorized that the very fragrant Old Garden roses with their beautiful petal-packed rosette-blooms and thorny stems have a healing signature that may directly correlate with the brain and

spinal cord of the human body. Perhaps the thorns, and even their arrangement on the stem (phylotaxis), correlate with the structure of the human central nervous system and specific nerve endings on the spinal column/spinal cord and meridians!

This information is intuitive, but within the science of herbal and flower essence therapy, which often associates physical characteristics of the individual flower and plant with aspects of human anatomy and personality, the possibility of this healing signature makes sense. A classic example of this in herbalism is how the ginseng root resembles a human form and is an effective tonic for the whole body.

I recently found the following information that seems to confirm my intuitions within this context:

> "...The cells of the brain and spinal cord, which frequently incur free radical damage, can be protected by significant amounts of vitamin C..." (J. Balch, M.D, P. Balch, CNC, *Prescription for Nutritional Healing, (Avery Penguin Putnam, 2000).*

Perhaps we have known this connection intuitively, as the rose is traditionally associated with the emotional and spiritual heart. Thus, the physical characteristics of the Old Garden roses seem to demonstrate the healing signature of the rose as it relates to human anatomy. With a little stretch of the imagination, one may see that the blooms and thorny stems of many of these roses remarkably resemble the human brain and spinal column, which are both protected by the Vitamin C found in rose hips! The flower essence made from the rose, stem and thorns, then, would vibrationally have a similar protective and nourishing/nurturing psycho-spiritual role for the individual.

Perhaps this could impact the practice of acupuncture, as the positions of thorns on the rose stem may correlate with specific acupuncture points associated with the spinal chord that stimulate certain nerve impulses affecting the brain and organs. Experiments with rose flower essences with spinal acupuncture may show us the effects of treatment with acupuncture needles dipped into specific rose flower essences and inserted into specific spinal points or direct application of the rose essences to corresponding acupuncture-meridian points without needles (floral acupressure).

Endnotes to Chapter Three

1. "Water's Energetic Nature" by Joshua Korn, Blend Magazine, Issue 77, pp. 72-3, Summer 2001.
2. "Water's Energetic Nature" by Joshua Korn, Blend Magazine, Issue 77, pp. 72-3, Summer 2001.
3. *The Message from Water*, pp. 127-8.
4. *The Healing Energies of Water*, p. 60.
5. *The Healing Energies of Water*, p. 66.
6. *The Healing Energies of Water*, p. 58.
7. In Succussion – The energy of a substance "...remains because each dilution is succussed, or shaken vigorously 100 times before proceeding to the next dilution. For instance, one drop from the mother tincture of a substance, added to 99 drops of water is succussed 100 times by striking the bottle against an object soft enough not to break the glass. This is a 1c potency, from which one drop is taken and added to 99 drops of water and succussed and properly diluted. Succussion may vary between remedies and production companies, but it is the movement of the liquid solution that establishes the breakdown of the molecules of each substance, not the type of succussion. The energy from the original substance remains in the diluted form of the remedy. This contains the essence of that substance, without any of its toxicity...In simplest terms, these are remedies because they resonate with the energetic pattern of the individual and stimulate a response from the vital force." [7] *Homeopathic Vibrations: A Guide for Natural Healing.*

Endnotes to Chapter Four

1. Stedman, Nancy, "Natural Havens," *Natural Health, July/August 2004, p. 64.*
2. Freeman, Ph.D., Victoria L., "Gardens: Nature's Health Source for Mind, Body & Spirit," *healthsmart today, Spring 2005, p. 62.*

Endnotes to Chapter Six

1. Matthew Ch. 6, v. 12, 14; Luke Ch.17, v. 3-4; Ch. 23, v. 34 *The Amplified Bible.*

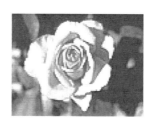

APPENDIX A
52 ROSES: COLOR, FRAGRANCE, AND BODY ENERGY CENTERS

Note: All roses correspond to the heart and crown of the head.

<u>Fragrance Key:</u>
Fr = Fruity
L = Light
M = Musky
NF = No Fragrance
P = Peppery
R = Rosy
Sp = Spicy
St = Strong
Sw = Sweet
T = Tea

<u>Body Energy Centers Key:</u>
R = Root (base of spine)
S = Sacrum
SP = Solar Plexus
H = Heart
T = Throat (front),
MO = Medulla Oblongata (base of skull)
B = Brow
C = Crown or Corona
MS= Mist Spray

ROSE VARIETY & FRAGRANCE	COLOR	BODY ENERGY CENTER
'Altissimo' (L)	Red	R * S * H* C * MS
'Anastasia' (L)	White	H * B * C * MS
'Arizona' (St)	Yellow/Orange	S * SP * H * C *MS
'Bill Warriner'(L)	Coral/Salmon Pink	S * SP * H * C * MS
'Bonica' (NF)	Pink	H * B * C * MS
'Brandy' (Fr, St, Sw)	Coral/Apricot	S * SP * H * C * MS
'Brass Band' (L)	Apricot/Pink	S * SP * H * C * MS
'Bride' (R)	Pink	R * H * C * MS
'Camara' (L)	Red	R * S * H * C * MS
'Cherish' (L)	Coral/Pink	S * SP * H * C * MS
'Chrysler Imperial' (St)	Red	R * S * H * C * MS
'Crystalline' (NF)	White	H * B * C * MS
'Double Delight' (Sp/Sw)	Pink/White	H * B * C * MS
'Eglantine' (St)	Pink	R * H * B * C * MS
'Electron' (St)	Electric Pink	R * H * B * C * MS

'Elizabeth Taylor' (Sp)	Pink	R * H * B * C * MS
'Evelyn' (St, Sw)	Apricot/Pink	S * SP * H * C * MS
'Fair Bianca' (St, Sw)	White	H * B * C * MS
'Fragrant Plum' (St, Sw)	Lavender/Purple	R * H * T * B * C * MS
'French Perfume' (R)	Cream Yellow/Pink	SP * H * C * MS
'Gertrude Jekyll' (St)	Deep Pink	R * H * C * MS
'Granada' (Sp, Sw)	Lt. Orange/Pink/ Yellow	S * SP * H * B * MS
'Grand Impression' (Fr)	Salmon/Yellow/ Apricot	S * SP * H * C * MS
'Guy de Maupassant'	Pink	R * H * C * MS
'Harlequin' (Sw)	Lavender/Mauve	H * T * B * C * MS
'Jayne Austin' (P)	Peach/Apricot	S * SP * H * C * MS
'Just Joey' (Fr, St)	Apricot	S * SP * H * C * MS
'LD Braithwaite' (St)	Red	R * S * H* MO *C * MS
'Lanvin' (St)	Yellow	S * SP * H * C * MS
'Louise Odier' (St)	Medium Pink	R * H * C * MS
'Melody Parfumee' (Sw, Sp)	Purple/Plum	R * H * T * B * C * MS
'Mister Lincoln' (R)	Red	R * S * H * C * MS

'Madame Isaac Pereire' (R, St)	Pink/Red/Purple	R * S * H * T * B * C * MS
'Mon Cheri' (L)	Deep Pink	R * H * C * MS
'Pat Austin' (Sw, T)	Yellow/Copper Orange	S * SP * H * C * MS
'Paul Shirville' (S)	Salmon/Pink	R * SP * H * B * C * MS
'Perdita' (L)	Apricot	S * SP * H * C * MS
'Pristine' (L)	White/tinged Pink	H * MO * B * C* MS
'Regatta' (Fr)	Pink/Peach	R * SP * H * T * C * MS
'Royal Dane' (Sw)	Pink/ Copper Orange	R * S * H * B * C * MS
'Royal Wedding' (St)	Apricot/Pink	R * S * H * C * MS
'Sea Pearl' (L)	Cream/Yellow/ Pink	S * SP * H * MO * C * MS
'Summer Fashion' (Fr)	Yellow/Pink	R * S * H * C * MS
'Summer's Kiss' (L)	Cream/Yellow	S * SP * H * C * MS
'Sunset Celebration' (Fr)	Apricot/Amber	S * SP * H * C * MS
'Tamora' (St)	Apricot/Yellow	S * SP * H * C * MS
'Tiffany' (Fr)	Lt. Pink/Yellow	S *SP * H * C * MS
'Timeless' (L)	Red	R * S * H * C * MS
'Tineke' (NF)	White/hint of Green	H * B * C * MS

'Touch of Class' (L)	Pink/Coral/Orange	R * S * H * C * MS
'Tournament of Roses' (L)	Coral/Pink	R * S * SP * H * C * MS
'Y'ves Piaget' (St)	Pink	R * H * C * MS

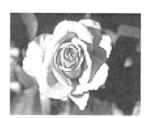

APPENDIX B
16 ROSES IN THE COMBINATION FORMULAS

'Altissimo' – *Stress Rescue* formula
'Anastasia' – *Lightness of Heart* formula
'Cherish' – *Share Love* formula
'Crystalline' – *Faith in the Storm* formula
'Double Delight' – *Grief Relief* formula
'Fair Bianca' – *Heart Balance, Stress Rescue* formulas
'Guy de Maupassant' – *Compassion ~ Forgiveness* formula
'Madame Isaac Pereire' – *Love Source* formula
'Pristine' – *Stress Rescue* formula
'Regatta' – *Stress Rescue* formula
'Sea Pearl' – *Self - Nurture* formula
'Summer Fashion' – *Stress Rescue* formula
'Tiffany' – *Self-Love & Peace* formula
'Timeless' – *Open Heart* formula
'Tineke' – *Loving Relationships* formula
'Y'ves Piaget' – *Grief Relief* formula

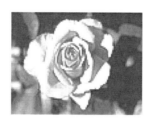

APPENDIX C
18 FLOWERS IN THE COMBINATION FORMULAS

Beech *(Fagus Grandifolia)* – Encourages compassion, tolerance and flexibility. *Compassion ~ Forgiveness* formula

Calendula (*Calendula Officinalis*) – Assists one in being more receptive and in listening without judging. *Self-Love & Peace* formula

Daffodil (*Narcissus Pseudonarcissus*) – Encourages self-esteem and acceptance. *Love's Expression* formula

Dandelion *(Taraxacum Officinale)* – Releases fear from the body, repressed emotions, tensions held in muscles and organs. Fosters courage and strength. *Stress Rescue* formula

Echinacea *(Echinacea Angustifolia)* – Helps to clear emotional blockages and to restore vital energy. *Love Source* formula

Harebell *(Mencopis Quintuplinervia)* – Encourages one to give and receive love unconditionally. *Loving Relationships* formula

Iris *(Iris Species)* – Helps to release creative blocks and feelings of limitation. Assists in finding meaning in life. *Self-Love & Peace* formula

Lilac *(Syringa Vulgaris)* – Enhances relaxation of the spine and flexibility. Expands intuitive states. *Compassion ~ Forgiveness* formula

Marigold *(see Calendula Oficinalis)* – Helps in hearing and understanding the truth of what is said. *Self-Love & Peace* formula

Mesquite *(Prosopis Torreyana, Prosopis Juliflora, Prosopis Alba)* – Brings abundance and pleasure. Amplifies compassion and warmth. *Open Heart* formula

Morning Glory *(Impomoea Purpurea)* – For loss of spiritual faith, addictions to opiates and nicotine. Helps break destructive habits. Balances nervous system. *Faith in the Storm* formula

Ocotillo *(Fouquieria Splendens)* – Encourages understanding and acceptance. Helps one in accepting and finding insight into subconscious or unexpressed emotions. *Grief Relief* formula

Primrose *(Primula Vulgaris)* – Brings lightness and openness and acceptance of love. *Love Source* formula

Rosemary *(Rosmarinus Officinalis)* – Offers strength to the heart and fosters trust. *Heart Balance* formula

Self-Heal *(Prunella Vulgaris)* – Assists one in trusting the process of healing. *Faith in the Storm* and *Stress Rescue* formulas

Shooting Star *(Dodecatheon clevelandii, Dodecatheon hendersonii, Dodecatheon pulchellum)* – Helps one to be less alienated and to be more caring and sharing of love. *Share Love*

Sweet White Violet *(Viola Blanda)* – Encourages openness, warmth and trust in one's interactions. *Heart Balance* formula

Zinnia *(Zinnia Elegans)* – Helps one to loosen up emotionally. Stimulates laughter, joy and cheerfulness as one re-connects with the child within. *Lightness of Heart* formula

APPENDIX D
ROSES FOR BALANCING ENERGY CENTERS

*O*ur bodies have centers of energy that correspond to specific organs, tissues, nerves and body systems. These centers interface between the physical, emotional, mental and spiritual aspects of our being. Each energy center filters energy from the environment around and within us and disperses it throughout our body. This energy is vital energy that helps to bring balance and vitality to the body. In the vibrational model, each energy center governs a gland in the physical body; corresponds to one of the seven colors of the rainbow and to a musical note in an octave; controls specific physical organs and aspects of our conscious awareness.

When the energies of the energy centers are flowing freely, we operate at our optimum level of physical, emotional and mental health. Rose flower essences can help to balance these centers of energy so that we can experience optimum health and wellbeing.

Root Center
Location: Base of spine (perineum)
Corresponding Color: Red
Corresponding Musical Note: C
Gland: Adrenals
Organs and Body Systems: Skeletal system, immune system, muscle tissue, legs and feet
Properties: Earth and nature connection, survival instinct; holds life force and when unbalanced we are ungrounded, spacey, neglectful of physical safety and health.

Roses for balancing: *'Altissimo', 'Bride', 'Camara', 'Chrysler Imperial', 'Double Delight', 'Eglantine', 'Electron', 'Elizabeth Taylor', 'Fragrant Plum', 'Gertrude Jekyll', 'Guy de Maupassant', 'LD Braithwaite', 'Louise Odier', 'Melody Parfumee', 'Mister Lincoln', 'Madame Isaac Pereire', 'Mon Cherie', 'Paul Shirville', 'Regatta', 'Royal Dane', 'Royal Wedding', 'Summer Fashion', 'Tiffany', 'Timeless', 'Touch of Class', 'Tournament of Roses', 'Y'ves Piaget'*

Sacral Center (Sacrum)

Location: Lower abdomen between ovaries in women and one inch below the navel in men, two inches into the body
Corresponding Color: Orange
Corresponding Musical Note: D
Gland: Spleen, gonads, and ovaries
Organs and Body Systems: Kidneys, bladder, genitals, uterus, ovaries and testes
Properties: Center of creativity and sexuality; governs passion, life pleasures, desires; when unbalanced we deny our desires, pleasure, and stifle our passion and creativity.
Roses for balancing: *'Altissimo'. 'Arizona', 'Bill Warriner', 'Brandy', 'Brass Band', 'Camara', Chrysler Imperial', 'Evelyn', 'Granada', 'Grand Impression', 'Jayne Austin', 'Just Joey', 'LD Braithwaite', 'Lanvin', 'Mister Lincoln', 'Madame Isaac Pereire', 'Pat Austin', 'Paul Shirville', 'Perdita', 'Regatta', 'Royal Dane', 'Royal Wedding', 'Sea Pearl', 'Summer Fashion', 'Summer's Kiss', 'Sunset Celebration', 'Tamora', 'Tiffany', 'Timeless', 'Touch of Class', 'Tournament of Roses'*

Solar Plexus Center

Location: Solar plexus, one inch above the navel at the nerve ganglion and over the stomach
Corresponding Color: Yellow
Corresponding Musical Note: E
Gland: Pancreas
Organs and Body Systems: Digestive system
Properties: Personal power, sense of place in the world, confidence, self-worth and ability to accept self-responsibility; when unbalanced addictions, excess self-criticism and control issues manifest.

Roses for balancing: *'Arizona', 'Bill Warriner', 'Brandy', 'Brass Band', 'Cherish', 'Evelyn', 'French Perfume', 'Granada', 'Grand Impression', 'Jayne Austin', 'Just Joey', 'Lanvin', 'Pat Austin', 'Paul Shirville', 'Perdita', 'Regatta', 'Sea Pearl', 'Summer's Kiss', 'Sunset Celebration', 'Tamora', 'Tiffany', 'Touch of Class', 'Tournament of Roses'*

Heart Center
Location: At the level of the heart (slightly right of the center of chest), between the shoulder blades (back)
Corresponding Color: Green, pink
Corresponding Musical Note: F
Gland: Thymus
Organs and Body Systems: Lungs, heart
Properties: Governs self-love and love for others, understanding, harmony, balance of the masculine and feminine aspects of self
Roses for balancing: *All Roses*

Heart-Thymus Center
Location: Between the heart and throat in the center of the chest
Corresponding Color: Light blue
Corresponding Musical Note: F#
Gland: Thymus
Properties: Seat of unconditional love, compassion, harmony and peace; when unbalanced we are non-empathetic, uncompassionate, unable to give and receive love.
Roses for balancing: *All Roses*

Throat Center
Location: Base of the throat (front), medulla oblongata - base of skull (back)
Corresponding Color: Blue
Corresponding Musical Note: G
Gland: Thyroid
Organs and Body Systems: Neck, shoulders and arms
Properties: Governs expression and thoughtful communication; hearing of the wise inner voice (conscience); ability to express truthfully; when out of balance, we may be over- or under-communicative, speak untruths or tell "little white lies".

Roses for balancing: *'Fragrant Plum', 'Harlequin', 'Melody Parfumee', 'Madame Isaac Pereire'*

Brow Center
Location: Center of forehead between the eyebrows
Corresponding Color: Purple, violet or indigo (blue-violet)
Corresponding Musical Note: A
Gland: Pineal
Organs and Body Systems: Eyes, sinuses
Properties: Governs insight, inner knowing (intuition) and imagination. An imbalance in this area may indicate disorientation, narrow-mindedness, being caught up in the "psychic" realm.
Roses for balancing: *'Anastasia', 'Bonica', 'Crystalline', 'Double Delight', 'Eglantine', 'Electron', 'Elizabeth Taylor', 'Fair Bianca', 'Fragrant Plum', 'Harlequin', 'Melody Parfumee', 'Madame Isaac Pereire', 'Pristine', 'Teneke'*

Crown or Corona
Location: Top of the head
Corresponding Color: Violet, Golden White
Corresponding Musical Note: B
Gland: Pituitary
Organs and Body Systems: Central nervous system
Properties: Governs connection with the divine; center of pure knowing and spiritual relationship; self-realization and unlimited potential; highest levels of consciousness.
Roses for balancing: *All Roses, especially 'Anastasia', 'Chrystalline', 'Double Delight', 'Fair Bianca', 'French Perfume', 'Pristine', 'Tineke'*

APPENDIX E
A TRANSCRIPT OF TWO BIOFEEDBACK
IMAGING SESSIONS

Session #1 – Donna, biofeedback imaging specialist, administers the unknown essence to author.
Before the essence is administered
T – O.K. – Testing, One, Two, Three, Four, Five, Six….
It's open.
Donna administers the essence, 'Fair Bianca'. *Tenanche closes her eyes. After about ninety seconds:*
T – That's my brain working still. I'm a very brainy person…
T- Look at my heart center. I really have to work on that! There's some grief there. Some grief comes up…
D – It's changed. There's a lot of pink over there.
 - A lot of blue. It's expressing the inner voice. Yeah, there's a lot of blue.

'Fair Bianca' rose flower essence administered to Tenanche by Donna
Bio-energy field is moving to magenta. Tenanche closes her eyes. It takes about three minutes for a visible change in the energy field to be recorded.
T – Still a lot of blue.
D – It is wonderful!
T – Where's all this pink coming from? Wow. This is **'Fair Bianca'** rose (she discovers, picking up the bottle). That pink there – we went from blue to indigo to pink.
D – I don't see very many like this!
T – This is so exciting for me! This is what I've dreamed of! It's great – and this one is pretty even…

D – Wow!

T – Look at that! Perfect! Perfect! All of the magenta emanating in the energy field…

Session #2 – Author administers essences to Marilyn.

Before essence is administered

T – O.K. This is Marilyn. Yaay!

M – Hi Mom!

T – As she arrived – lots of blue, green, and white – love energy…

M – I've got shoes on. Should I take them off?

T – Well, for you – yeah!

Her energy field jumps on the video and printout.

T – Wow! Look at that! That's incredible! A huge white light at the crown opened up and the heart opened up a lot

T – Marilyn is so open and sensitive to our stone friends. They're in the whole room

M – It is kind of too late now.

Author moves the essence bottles further away from Marilyn, who is extremely sensitive to the vibrations of the essences. Author administers the next essence, 'Fair Bianca', under the tongue and at the nape of the neck. Marilyn closes her eyes.

M – Um, I like that.

T – This is essence number one – four drops under the tongue as well as a drop at the base of the neck. (*Marilyn closes her eyes*).

M – Well, there's certain moments where things flash in. What I felt was an inverted triangle – lower point at solar plexus. (*Ninety seconds pass*).

T – This is **'Fair Bianca'** rose.

M – My birth flower is the rose, so I may feel it very specifically.

T – Her birth flower is the rose. Let's meditate on this and I'm sure more will come. (*The image is printed out*).

T – More violet around the edges…looking at the heart – There's more white there. A little bit more white at the crown there also. O.K….

M – Like, I feel like that little bird. That's sort of what it reminds me of.

Marilyn is inspired and shares a couple of her humorous anecdotes with us for a few minutes. Author administers the next essence, *Stress Rescue Formula* under the tongue and a few drops at the base of the spine.

M – Oh, man… (*She closes her eyes*) Oh, wow… image is yellow…
T – That's your brain.
M – It shot right up there immediately. It felt like it was going to come off!
T – Really! That is the last one. It has four roses. I call it *Stress Rescue*. Maybe it's too much. You said that it shot right up…
M – Yeah. Well, it shot up – but it didn't stay there. But now I'm here. I felt that one more that any of them…Good rocket ride.
T – Oh, more green in there!
M – What I need to do next…
D – The heart is more open.
T – The heart is more open and there's more green there.
D – There's a lot more down here… at the base of the spine.
T – Maybe there's a little bit more at the brow…
M – Yeah.
T – Thank you so much!
M – This was fun!

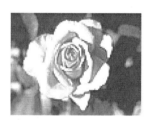

GLOSSARY OF ROSE CATEGORIES

Bourbon Rose – An Old Garden Rose that originated on the island in the Indian Ocean known as L'lle de Bourbon (now Reunion Island). A vigorous, hardy, compact, shrub that is useful as a hedge.

Damask Rose – A species rose that dates all the way back to early Greek civilization. Very hardy, especially in cold winters. Extremely fragrant, very thorny, and blooms once a year.

Floribunda Rose – A free and prolific blooming shrub that produces dozens of flowers that bloom in clusters or *sprays*. A favorite rose for landscaping.

Grandiflora Rose – A tall, vigorous bush that forms beautiful large hybrid tea-like blooms and long stems, which grow in clusters. Sometimes the blooms come one to a stem, as do hybrid teas.

Hybrid Tea Rose – The most popular type of rose sold in flower shops and possibly the most popular flower in the world. It is usually a plant with long, open canes. It has beautiful long-stemmed flowers of up to 60 or more petals that can be 5 inches wide, which bloom repeatedly during the season. They are ideal for cutting.

Old Garden Rose or English Rose – Also referred to as an *antique rose;* this rose preceded modern varieties that originated in the 20th century. It is a bush or shrub rose that falls within the category of a large group of roses whose parentage includes species roses. This type of rose precedes the modern hybrid tea rose and tends to be intensely fragrant with dozens of petals on each bloom.

Shrub Rose – A rose that grows as a bush and can be pruned and cut to form shrubbery.

Species or Wild Rose – The 5-petaled parent or ancestor roses from which all hybridized roses descend. Two species roses are Dog Rose (*Rosa canina*) and Damask Rose (*Rosa damascena*).

Glossary of Terms

Acupuncture – An ancient method of therapy and pain relief that involves puncturing specific sites of the body with needles.

Adoration – An act of adoring or worshipping.

Alignment – The condition of being in satisfactory adjustment or having the parts in proper relative position to one another.

Angel – A divine being; a messenger of God.

Aromatherapy – The art and science of using plant oils in treatment and therapy.

Aspiration – A desire or ambition.

Attune, attunement – To harmonize with; the state of being in harmony with a specific spiritual quality.

Ayurveda – A traditional East Indian system of medicine based largely on homeopathy and natural healing.

Bach Flower Remedies – A healing system of using the vibrational essences of 38 wildflowers for physical, emotional, spiritual and healing, developed in the 1930s by British physician, Dr. Edward Bach.

Bio-energetic System – A system of the body that includes both the human biological and subtle energy systems.

Biofeedback Imaging Photography/Video – An interactive multi-media biofeedback technology that measures, analyzes and interprets human emotional-energetic activity and displays it in photo and/or video form.

Calibrate – To rectify or correct to a certain measurement or frequency.

Catalyze – To cause.

Celestial – To be heavenly; Divine.

Christ (The Anointed One) – Jesus (Yeshua), The Son of God; The Anointed One; The Messiah; God Incarnate, "The Rose of Sharon".

Clustered Water™ – Pure water whose inherent natural structure remains intact, unlike tap or piped water which lacks one electron from its outer orbit; brand name of structured water distributed by Cellcore International, Inc.

Compassion – The spiritual consciousness of the suffering of others and directing selfless tenderness toward it.

Consciousness – The awareness of one's existence, feelings and thoughts.

Contemplate – To reflect deeply upon.

Cranial-Sacral (Craniosacral) Therapy – A therapy originated in 1901 by Dr. William Sutherland, D.O. in which imbalances in the body are perceived via the motion of the cranial bones which are then manipulated to help re-establish harmony.

Cultivar, Cultivated (rose) – A variety that has originated and persisted under cultivation.

Devotion – A spiritual affection, love or zeal.

Dilution – Resulting from the addition of water to change the strength of a substance.

Dimension – A plane of existence.

Divine – Concerned with the sacred; emanating from God.

Divine Grace – Beneficence or generosity shown or given to humans by God.

Doctrine of Signature – The principle that there is a direct relationship between the physical human body and the physical, chemical attributes of plants, minerals and other healing agents.

Dosage Essence – The essence of a flower arrived at by diluting the stock essence in a specific manner so that it may be administered in precise doses.

Essence – The basic underlying substance, form or energy of a thing.

Ether – The rarified element of the heavens; a medium that permeates all space and transmits waves of energy; the realm where energy lives and weaves itself.

Evolution – The process of change, unfolding, movement, progressive development and transformation.

Expansion – The process of spreading out; increasing, growing, amplifying.

Faith – Belief without proof; confidence or reliance.

Flavenoid – A nutrient that supports the function of the body's immune system.

Forgive – To cease to feel resentment toward on account of a wrong committed and to give up claim to seek retribution; to unconditionally absolve or pardon.

Frequency – A vibration or energy wave.

Gratitude – Thankfulness.

HADO – a Japanese term for the intrinsic vibrational pattern or vital energy of a substance or body

Halo – A zone of light surrounding a central body.

Harmonize – To bring into harmony or agreement.

Healing – The act of restoring health and balance.

Herbalism or Herbology – The medicinal use of herbs for healing.

Higher Purpose – A purpose set forth from God.

Homeopath – A licensed practitioner of homeopathy.

Homeopathy – A complete system of healing developed by German physician Samuel Hahnemann that is based on the principle of "like cures like"– that a natural substance that can cause disease in a healthy person, when used in dilute quantities can relieve the same disease and restore health.

Hybrid, Hybridized Rose – A rose whose parents are two different varieties.

Immune System – The system of the physical body that protects it from invading organisms and disease.

Infinite Source – God: The Ineffable Beginning of All Things.

Infusion – The liquid that results from the steeping or soaking of a substance (mineral or flower) in water in order to extract its virtues for healing.

Innate – To be inherent; to be natural.

Intuition – A knowing or perception by intuition or direct insight.

Kinesiology – A study of and use of the principles of mechanics and anatomy in relation to human movement.

LaStone Therapy™ – A system of healing massage developed by Mary Nelson that alternates the use of hot and cold, river rocks utilizing massage techniques to assist the body in releasing blockages and to accelerate healing.

Light – The spiritual illumination that is a divine attribute or the embodiment of divine truth; the underlying essential composing element of space and the cosmos, of which visible light is a manifestation.

Lycopene – A substance, similar to carotene, which gives tomatoes, berries and rose hips their red coloring.

Massage Therapy – The manipulation of body tissues by stroking, kneading, and tapping to improve muscle tone, circulation, reduce muscle tension, stress, and to prevent disease and restore health.

Meditate – To contemplate; to clear the mind of everyday worries and concerns.

Meditation – A state of contemplation.

Meridians – Patterns of energy flow that carry vital or life force into and throughout the physical body.

Mother Essence – The original essence of a flower blossom imprinted in pure water that is preserved for further dilution as a stock or dosage essence.

Muse – The creative spirit of an individual.

Nature – The created earth in its natural state.

Neuro-Emotional Release Therapy or Neuro-Emotional Technique (N.E.T.) – A physiological treatment using structural manipulation that can help to normalize neurological imbalance, remove emotional blocks and reduce stress in the body, offered by holistic physicians and chiropractors.

Paradigm – An example or pattern.

Potentize – To make more potent or effective.

Prayer – A humble approach to God in word, thought, petition, praise, devotion, worship, adoration or thanksgiving.

Psycho-spiritual – Relating to both the psyche (personality) and the spirit.

Radiance – A vivid brightness; a splendor of light.

Ray – A beam of light or other radiant energy.

Realm – Region, territory, domain or kingdom.

Red Shiso – An herbal extract that is sometimes used as a preservative or stabilizer in making flower essences. Its Latin name is *Perilla frutescens*. Known for its red color, this member of the mint family contains perilla aldehyde, a preservative that is 1000 times stronger than synthetic food preservatives. It is used in Japan for seasoning, coloring and pickling foods. In Chinese medicine it is considered a warming herb that calms the nervous system. It has a strong, pungent flavor.

Reflexology – A healing science based upon the principle that reflex areas in the feet and hands correspond to all glands, organs and parts of the body. Proper stimulation of these reflex areas encourages the body's natural healing response.

Rose Hip – The seedpod that remains when the flower's petals fall off that is full of seeds high in Vitamin C content.

Resonate – To vibrate sympathetically.

Rosette – A cluster of petals or leaves arranged in a circular pattern.

Service – To act for the benefit of others without seeking compensation or self-benefit.

Somatic Therapy – A category of several types of therapy that encourage the healing of imbalances in the body through awareness and movement. Dance Movement Therapy and Feldenkrais™ are two somatic therapies.

Soul – A person's mind, will and emotions.

Soul Quality – A characteristic of the soul differentiated from that of the personality.

Spirit – The breath of life; the animating or vital life-giving principle of living organisms.

Spiritual – Relating to the spirit, rather than to the physical; sacred, holy or divine.

Stock Essence – The first generation dilution of the mother essence.

Succussion – The shaking of a substance (usually a homeopathic remedy) in order to release kinetic energy from the mass of the substance into water.

Surrender – To relinquish power, control or authority.

Synchronize – To cause to coincide or co-exist.

Tincture – A quintessential active alchemical substance capable of causing physical, mental or emotional changes.

Toxicologist – A specialist who deals with toxic substances and their effects on living organisms.

Transform – To change in character, condition or function; to change in outward appearance or form.

Universe, Universal – Cosmic; pertaining to the whole cosmos rather than merely the earth.

Vegan – A vegetarian who consumes no food derived from animals, dairy, fowl or insects.

Vegetable Glycerin – A sweet, syrupy trihydroxy alcohol obtained by saponification of vegetable oil. It can be used as a preservative and stabilizer for flower essences.

Vegetarian – A person whose diet omits animal flesh.

Vibration – A characteristic emanation of energy that infuses or vitalizes.

Vibrational Medicine, Energy Medicine – A field of medicine based upon the study of subtle energies and their effects on the human bio-energetic system.

REFERENCES

Books

Balch, J., M.D., and Phyllis A., C.N.C. *Prescription for Nutritional Healing: A Practical A-Z Reference to Drug-Free Remedies Using Vitamins, Minerals, Herbs and Food Supplements, 3rd Edition.* New York, NY: Avery Penguin Putnam, 2000.

Ball, Stefan. *Bach Flower Remedies.* Chicago, IL: Teach Yourself Books, 2000.

Barnard, Julian & Martine. *The Healing Herbs of Edward Bach: An Illustrated Guide to the Flower Remedies.* Bath, England: Ashgrove Press Limited, 1995.

Barrett, Ph.D., Marilyn. *Creating Eden: The Garden as a Healing Space.* New York: HarperCollins, 1992.

Brennan, Georgeanne. *Easy Roses: Simple Secrets for Glorious Gardens, Indoors and Out.* San Francisco: Chronicle Books, 1995.

Chancellor, Dr. Philip M. *Handbook of the Bach Flower Remedies.* London: Keats Publishing, 1971.

Dancu, David A., N.D. *Homeopathic Vibrations: A Guide for Natural Healing.* Hygiene, CO: Sunshine Press Publications, 1996.

Davis, Patricia. *An A-Z Aromatherapy.* Essex, U.K.: C.W. Daniel Company, Ltd., 1999.

Emoto, Masaru. *The Message from Water, Vols. 1, 2, and 3*. Tokyo, JAPAN: Hado Publishing, 2001-2004.

Erasmus, Udo. *Fats that Heal, Fats that Kill: The Complete Guide to Fats, Oils, Cholesterol and Human Health.* Burnaby, B.C.: Alive Books, 1993.

Gerber, M.D., Richard. *Vibrational Medicine: New Choices for Healing Ourselves.* Santa Fe, NM: Bear and Company, 1988.

Griffiths, Trevor. *The Book of Old Roses.* London: Mermaid Books, 1984.

Harvey, Clare G., Cochrane, Amanda. *The Encyclopaedia of Flower Remedies.* San Francisco, CA: Thorsons, 1995.

Heinerman, John. *Healing Herbs and Spices.* Paramus, NJ: Parker Publishing Company - Prentice Hall, 1996.

Lawless, Julia. *Rose Oil: A New Guide to Nature's Most Precious Perfume and Traditional Remedies.* London: Thorson's, 1995.

Lazzara, Margó Valentine, C.Ht. *The Healing Aromatherapy Bath: Therapeutic Treatments Using Meditation, Visualization & Essential Oils.* Pownal, VT: Storey Books, 1999.

Mattock, J., et al. *The Complete Book of Roses.* London: Ward Lock Limited, 1994.

McDonald, Elvin. *Tea Roses.* New York, NY: Smithmark Publishers, 1998.

Ryrie, Charlie. *The Healing Energies of Water.* Boston, MA: Journey Editions, 1999.

Scarman, John. *Gardening with Old Roses.* New York, NY: Harper Collins, 1996.

Utterback, C., Ruggiero, M. *The Serious Gardener™ Reliable Roses: The New York Botanical Garden.* New York, NY: Clarkson Potter, 1997.

Walheim, Lance, et al. *Roses for Dummies, 2nd Edition.* Foster City, CA: IDG Books Worldwide, Inc., 2000.

Weeks, Nora. *The Medical Discoveries of Edward Bach, Physician.* New Canaan, CT: Keats Publishing, 1994.

Worwood, Valerie Ann. *The Fragrant Heavens: the spiritual dimension of fragrance and aromatherapy.* Novato, California: New World Library, 1999.

_____, *Taylor's Guide to Roses* (Based on Taylor's Encyclopedia of Gardening, Fourth Edition.) Boston, MA: Houghton Mifflin Company, 1986.

The Amplified Bible, Expanded Edition. Grand Rapids, MI: Zondervan, 1987.

Articles in Journals and Magazines

Barnao, Vasudeva. "The Wildflowers of Australia – Living Essences of Australia" *Essences of Nature Magazine*, Vol. 3, Issue 3, pp. 26.

Berkowsky, B. "The Soul Nature of Rose Oil", *Massage and Bodywork*, June/July 2002, p. 55.
Freeman, Ph.D., Victoria L. "Gardens: Nature's Health Source for Mind, Body & Spirit," *healthssmart today,* Spring 2005, pp. 60-65.

Olympian Labs, Inc., Product Reference Guide, 2002.

Korn, Joshua. "Water's Energetic Nature", *Magical Blend Magazine,* Issue 77, Summer 2001, pp. 72-73.

Stedman, Nancy. "Natural Havens", *Natural Health,* July/August 2004, pp. 63-69.

Nature Biotechnology, September 2001; 19: 823-24, pp. 833-837.

World Wide Web

www.dictionary.com - On-Line Reference Dictionary
www.backyardgardener.com/masterg/rosehips.html -
Dr. Leonard Perry, "Rose Hips".
www.essences.com - *The World Wide Essence Society* website
www.hado.net *HADO – The Messages from Water* website of
Dr. Masaru Emoto
www.lef.org/magazine/mag99/aug99-report1.htm - T. Mitchell, "Lycopene: The Rediscovered Carotene," Life Extension Magazine, Aug. 1999.
www.rlrouse.com/rose-hips.html - "Growing and Harvesting Rose Hips"
www.rosaflora.net - *Rosaflora Flower Essences* website

HEALING THERAPIES CONTACT INFORMATION

Use this list to find qualified practitioners and/or training programs for the therapies mentioned in this book that can be complementary to your personal healing program with rose flower essences.

Acupuncture
Acupuncture and Oriental Medicine Alliance (AOMA)
14637 Starr Road SE
Olalla, WA 98359
Ph: 253.851.6896
Fax: 253.851.6883
E-Mail: info@www.AcupunctureAlliance.org
Website: www.AcupunctureAlliance.org

Aromatherapy
American Aromatherapy Association
P.O. Box 1222
Fair Oaks, CA 95628

International Aromatherapy and Herb Association
3541 West Acapulco Lane
Phoenix, AZ 85053
Ph: 602.938.4439
Website: www.aztecfreenet.org/iaha

International Federation of Aromatherapists
Stanford House
2-4 Chiswick High Road
London, W4 1TH
ENGLAND

National Association for Holistic Aromatherapy
219 Carl Street
San Francisco, CA 94117
Toll-Free: 888.ASKNAHA
Ph: 206.547.2164
Fax: 206.547.2680
E-Mail: info@naha.org
Website: www.naha.org

Biofeedback Imaging Photography and Video
Inneractive Enterprises, Inc.
4051 Glencoe, Suite 10
Venice, CA 90292
Ph: 310.578.5810
Fax: 310.578.5480
E-Mail: aura@inneractive.com
Website: www.inneractive.com

Bach Flower Therapy
Dr. Edward Bach Centre
Mount Vernon, Bakers Lane
Sotwell, Oxon, OXIO OPZ
U.K.
Ph: +44 (0) 149.1.8314678
Fax: +44 (0) 1491.825022
Website: www.bachcentre.com

Nelson Bach USA, Ltd.
Wilmington, MA 01887
Toll-Free: 800.319.9151
Ph: 1.978.988.3833
Fax: 1.978.988.1233

Clustered Water™
Abanero, LLC
420 Decatur St. SW
Olympia, WA 98502
Ph: 360.438.0143
Fax: 360.491.1866
Website: www.clusteredwateronline.com

Cellcore International
Ph: 480.964.1125

Cranial-Sacral Therapy
International School for Biodynamic Cranial-Sacral Therapy
P.O. Box 14760
North Palm Beach, FL 33408
Ph: 561.863.3350
Fax: 561.863.4409
E-Mail: info@sheacranial.com
Website: www.sheacranial.com

Flower Essence Research and Therapy
Flower Essence Society (FES)
P.O. Box 459
Nevada City, CA 95959
Toll-Free: 800.736.9222
Ph: 530.265.9163
Fax: 530.265.0584
E-Mail: mail@flowersociety.org
Website: www.flowersociety.org

International Healing Rose Society (IHRS)
c/o Rosaflora Botanicals
P.O. Box 91104
Pittsburgh, PA 15221
412.244.7788
E-Mail: healingrose@rosaflora.net
Website: www.rosaflora.net/healingrose

World Wide Essence Society (WWES)
P.O. Box 285
Concord, MA 01742
Ph: 978.369.8454
E-Mail: wwes@essences.com
Website: www.essences.com

Herbalism, Herbology
Herbalgram: The Journal of the American Botanical Council
6200 Manor Rd.
Austin, TX 78723
Ph: 512.922.4900
Fax: 512.926.2345
E-Mail: abc@herbalgram.org
Website: www.herbalgram.org

Journal of Medical Herbalism
Bergner Communication
P.O. Box 20512
Boulder, CO 80328
Website: www.medherb.com

Homeopathy
National Center for Homeopathy (NCH)
801 N. Fairfax St.
Suite 306
Alexandria, VA 22314
Toll-Free: 877.624.0613
Ph: 703.548.7790
Fax: 703.548.7792
Website: www.homeopathic.org

Alliance of Registered Homeopaths (ARH)
26 Sunningdale Ave.
Leigh-on-Sea
Essex SS91JZ
U.K.
Ph/Fax: 0800.736339

Ørjan Repaal
ABC klinikken
Alternativ Behandling Center
Holmenveien 1, Vinderen, 0374
Oslo, NORWAY
Ph: 97.54.64.03
E-Mail: homotoxolog@tiscali.no

Kinesiology (Applied Kinesiology)
International College of Applied Kinesiology (ICAK)
ICAK-USA
6405 Metcalf Ave., Ste. 503
Shawnee Mission, KS 66202
Ph: 913.384.5336
Fax: 913.384.5112
E-Mail: icakusa@usa.net
Website: www.icakusa.com

LaStone Therapy™
LaStone Therapy™ Center
2979 E. Broadway Blvd. Suite 224
Tucson, AZ 85716
Ph: 520.319.6414
Fax; 520.319.6415
E-Mail: info@lastonetherapy.com
Website: www.lastonetherapy.com

Massage Therapy
American Massage Therapy Association (AMTA)
820 Davis St.
Evanston, IL 60201
Website: www.amtamassage.org

Desert Institute of Healing Arts (DIHA)
(Specializing in Massage Therapy and Zen Shiatsu)
639 N. Sixth Avenue
Tucson, AZ 85705
Toll-Free: 800.733.8098
Ph: 520.882.0899
Website: www.desertinstitute.org

Finger Lakes School of Massage (FLSM)
1251 Trumansburg Road
Itaca, NY 14850
Ph: 607.272.9024
Fax: 607.272.4271
Website: www.flsm.com

**Neuro-Emotional Release Therapy or
Neuro-Emotional Technique (N.E.T.)**
Scott Walker, D.C., (Founder)
520 Second Street
Encintas, CA 92024
Toll-Free: 800.888.4638
Ph. 760.944.1030
Website: www.netmindbody.com

Reflexology
The International Institute of Reflexology, Inc.
5650 Fifth Avenue North
P.O. Box 12642
St. Petersburg, FL 33733-2642
Ph: 727.343.4811
Fax: 727.381.2807
E-Mail: iir@tampabay.rr.com
Website: www.reflexology-usa.net

Somatic Therapy
International Somatic Movement Education & Therapy
Association (ISMETA)
P.O. box 547
Hadley, MA 01035
Ph: 212.229.7666
E-Mail: info@ismeta.org

Veganism, Vegetarianism
The Vegetarian Resource Group
P.O. Box 1463
Baltimore, MD 21203
Ph: 410.366.VEGE

E-Mail: vrg@vrg.org
Website: www.vrg.org

Internet Resources
Healing Gardens Information
www.healinglandscapes.org
www.dirtworks.us
www.labyrinthsociety.org

Organic Gardening
www.organicgardening.com
www.homeharvest.com/linksorganic.htm
www.goingorganic.com
www.composters.com

Organic Nurseries
www.GardensAlive.com
www.plantideas.com/rose/index.html

Rose Resources (General)
www.EveryRose.com
www.FindMyRoses.com
www.HelpMeFindRoses.com
www.rosemania.com
www.yesterdaysroses.com

Resources for Amber and Cobalt Glass Bottles
www.burchbottle.com
www.libertynatural.com
www.sunburstbottle.com

Resource for Violet Glass Bottles
Miron Glass USA
2485 N. Beachwwod Drive
Los Angeles, CA 90068
Ph/Fax: 323.467-0558
E-Mail: mironusa@aol.com
Website: www.miron.ch (In German)

Resources for Pure Organic Essential Oils, Rosewater and Hydrosols
www.frontiercoop.com
www.lavenderlane.com
www.libertynatural.com
www.therapeuticgradeessentialoils.com

Resources for Red Shiso (*Red Shiso Perilla Frutescens*)
www.BloomsForLess.com
http://kitazawaseed.com/seeds_perilla.html
www.treefrogfarm.com

Sources for Massage/Reflexology Stones
www.akobi.com
www.lastonetherapy.com

AFTERWORD

*A*ll the work and research with these rose flower essences has been carried out without grants or financial support. Most of the anecdotal information has been gleaned from healing practitioners and lay people who have requested and documented use of the essences via my Rose Essence Research Program. The purpose of this ongoing program is to gather, research and disseminate information to the flower essence community and the general public about the healing potentials of rose flower essences.

If you would like to provide information, monetary support to assist with this research, or would like to order more copies of this book, please contact the author. In advance, I thank you for your generous support.

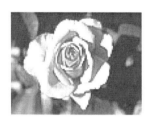

INDEX

information
    transmission of biological, 14
    electromagnetic, 14
    HADO, 14
    water retains and transmits, 15
inner conflict, 22
    knowing, 150
    strength, 128
    voice, hear, 65, 69, 149, 151
innocence, 20, 32, 54, 65, 81
insight, 37, 48, 146
    spiritual, 83, 85
insincere, 62
inspiration, xvi, 23, 40
    divine, 99
    cards, 179
integrity, 87, 131
intellect, 54, 55, 103, 126, 128
intellectual method of choosing essences, 77
intuition, 19, 103, 107, 133, 150, 159
inventor, 41, 81, 85
Iris flower *(Iris Species)*, 63, 145
isolation, 53

Jasmine *(Jasminum officinale, J. grandiflorum, J. sambac)*, 98, 99, 100
'Jayne Austin', 20, 32, 80, 84, 139, 148, 149
journey, spiritual, 25
joy, xv, 10, 11, 21, 32, 81, 84, 85, 107, 108, 146
    cultivate, 8, 18
    embrace, 51
    inspire, 40, 43
    lose touch with, 65
    radiance of, 24
    receive, 43
    support, 33
joyful, 55, 112, 129
judgment, 67, 68, 103, 145
'Just Joey', 32, 84, 139, 148, 149

kidneys, 7, 102, 148
kinesiology, using to choose essences, 4, 75–76, 111, 112, 159, 171

overwhelmed, 104, 110, 118, 119

pain, 9, 52, 65, 74, 104
    back, 110
    emotional, 9
    muscle, 109
    relief, 157
    unresolved, 105
    soothe, 98
    stomach, 75
painful times, 11
passion, 5, 148
past, letting go of, 51
    living in, 50
    stuck in, 52
'Pat Austin', 36, 85, 110, 112, 140, 148, 149
patience, 10, 43, 72, 82, 85, 91
pattern of imbalance, 47, 48, 50, 53, 56, 58, 61, 63, 66, 67, 77
'Paul Shirville', 36, 80, 82, 85,140, 148, 149
peace, 18, 22, 62, 64, 79, 84, 120, 128, 129, 149
    inner, 63
peaceful, 17, 64, 80, 82, 84, 120
    cooperation, 28
    mind, 119
perception, 159
    heightened, 37, 82, 85
'Perdita', 37, 80, 81, 85, 140, 148, 149
perfectionism, 61, 66
perseverance, 5, 39, 82, 85
Persians, and roses, 5
persona, false, 74
personal power, 148
personality, 133, 160, 161
    creative, 128
    false, 74
    fragmented, 10
    imbalances, xvi, 7
    injured, 9
    resignation in, 8
    reharmonize, 10
Philia, 11

vegan, 162, 172
vegetable glycerine, 94, 162
vegetarian, 162, 172
vibration, 52, 58, 65, 152, 159
    healing, 6
Vibration Magazine, 181
vibrational container, quartz as, 88
    difference, 123
    essences, 157, 181
    healing, 13
    medicine, 162
    memory, 15, 92
    model, 147
    remedies, 107
victim role, 61
vinegar as a preservative, 92, 93
visualize, 24, 72, 73
vital energy, 69, 147, 159
    increase, 127
    restore, 58, 145
Vitamin C, xvii, 7, 9, 131, 132, 133, 161
vitality,
    bring to body, 147
vodka as a preservative, 92, 93, 94

water, memory of, xviii, 13–16
wellbeing, 17, 26, 83, 103, 128, 147
    increase, 1
White Violet flower (sweet) *(Viola Blanda),* 52, 146
Wild Rose, xv, 5, 6, 7, 8, 90, 156
will, self-, 47
World Wide Essence Society, 166, 170, 181
wonder, sense of, 32, 83, 84
work space, spray essence in, 25
worry, 55, 103, 118

Ylang Ylang *(Cananga odorata),* 98, 99
'Y'ves Piaget', 43, 50, 80, 81, 82, 85, 111, 112, 141, 143, 148

Zinnia flower *(Zinnia Elegans),* 54, 55, 146

CONTACT INFORMATION

Rosaflora Botanicals
Products and Services:
Rosaflora™ Flower Essences
Rose Flower Essence Aroma Mists
The Healing-Roses Inspiration Cards

Tenanche Rose Golden, M.A.
Flower Essence Therapy
Specializing in rose flower essences and combination formulas
Bach Flower Essences
Consultations
Classes, Workshops
Home Study Course

Rosaflora Botanicals
P.O. Box 91104
Pittsburgh, PA 15221, USA
Ph: 412.244.7788
E-Mail:
info@rosaflora.net

Websites:
www.rosaflora.net

The International Healing Rose Society
(IHRS)
and
Healing Rose Press
P.O. Box 91104
Pittsburgh, PA 15221
Ph: 412.244.7788
Website: www.rosaflora.net/healingrose

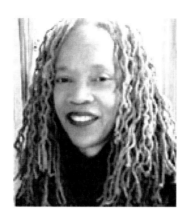

ABOUT THE AUTHOR

*T*enanche Rose Golden, M.A., R.M.T. is an experienced flower essence practitioner who has been using, researching and formulating vibrational essences since 1989. She has also studied Bach Flower Therapy with the British Institute of Homeopathy. The founder and former owner of Crystal Radiance Essences (mineral and flower essences), she is the owner of Rosaflora Botanicals and founder of Rosaflora Flower Essences. She now focuses exclusively on researching and formulating rose flower essences and educates others about their healing benefits.

Tenanche has written articles about rose flower essences for *Vibration Magazine* of the World Wide Essence Society, the *LaStone Therapy™ Newsletter* and *The Thrip Hater,* the Newsletter of the Rose Society of Tucson, among others. She is a member of the American Botanical Council, Flower Essence Society and National Gardening Association. Tenanche is the founder of the International Healing Rose Society, an association devoted to researching and educating about the therapeutic uses of roses and Healing Rose Press, a vehicle to publish this research.

A Reiki Master Practitioner and Teacher, reflexologist and artist, Tenanche is interested in documenting rose flower essence therapy in conjunction with Acupuncture, Massage, Reflexology and Art Therapy.

Give the Gift of Healing
With Rose Flower Essences
To Your Loved Ones, Friends, and Colleagues

CHECK LULU.COM, AMAZON.COM,
LOCAL BOOKSTORE OR ORDER HERE

YES, I want _____ copies of *Rose Flower Essences* at $18.95 each, plus $4 shipping per first book, $1.00 per additional book (PA residents please add $1.33 sales tax per book). Canadian orders must be accompanied by a postal money order in U.S. funds. International orders must be accompanied by a certified international check in U.S. funds. Allow 15-21 days for delivery.

My check or money order for $_____ is enclosed.

If you wish to pay by credit card, pay securely on our website at www.rosaflora.net

Name: _____

Organization: _____

Address: _____

City/State/Zip: _____

Phone: **Email:** _____

(Quantity Discounts Available)
Please make your check payable and return to:

Rosaflora Botanicals
P.O. Box 91104
Pittsburgh, PA 15221
Phone: 1-412-244-7788
Email: info@rosaflora.net

Made in United States
North Haven, CT
31 January 2023

31836894R00138